Menopause the Healthy, Happy Way

Menopause the Healthy, Happy Way

Nutrition for Change and Growth

María Tránsito López

Translated by Natalie Marie Linton

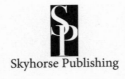

Skyhorse Publishing

All inquiries should be addressed to Skyhorse Publishing, 307 West 36th Street, 11th Floor, New York, NY 10018.

Skyhorse Publishing books may be purchased in bulk at special discounts for sales promotion, corporate gifts, fund-raising, or educational purposes. Special editions can also be created to specifications. For details, contact the Special Sales Department, Skyhorse Publishing, 307 West 36th Street, 11th Floor, New York, NY 10018 or info@skyhorsepublishing.com.

Skyhorse® and Skyhorse Publishing® are registered trademarks of Skyhorse Publishing, Inc.®, a Delaware corporation.

Visit our website at www.skyhorsepublishing.com.

10 9 8 7 6 5 4 3 2 1

Library of Congress Cataloging-in-Publication Data is available on file.

Cover design by Jane Sheppard
Cover photo credit: Dreamstime

Print ISBN: 978-1-5107-0555-5
Ebook ISBN: 978-1-5107-0560-9

Printed in the United States of America

For all women

TABLE OF CONTENTS

Introduction

Menopause is a completely normal physiological event that, sooner or later, will occur in the life of every woman. Therefore, and despite the pharmaceutical industry's intention to convert it into an unwanted disorder to be fixed with medication, it is not an illness.

Menopause opens the door to a new form of being and experiencing life, but, as in all periods of change, it is very probable that throughout its course various stressors arise, mainly because of the hormone imbalances that it will produce. However, once getting through this stage, the body will have achieved its new balance and, with it, the discomfort will disappear.

This being said, it is true that as a consequence of the most common lifestyle in our society, many women will suffer these symptoms with certain intensity and discomfort, causing them to seek alternatives to relieve them. But, before turning to pharmaceutical hormonal treatments that are usually proposed to alleviate these symptoms, it is essential to seek advice about what is going on and what options exist to improve the situation, and, once well-informed, reflect and decide.

Hormone Replacement Therapy (HRT) to treat symptoms of menopause is not necessarily free from side-effects and serious health-risks. In some very specific cases, it can be convenient, but, for the majority of women who have natural menopause with moderate symptoms, this treatment causes more harm than good.

Nevertheless, little interest in revealing other basic health information for women exists, in contrast to the great effort to promote this type of medicine. Yes, they should also communicate that our body, if we nurture it, train it, and let it rest as needed, is fully capable of combatting hormonal changes that take place in this stage. In other words, if we satisfy its demands and clean up our habits, our body has proper means to emerge successful and healthy from this journey.

Here is where this book intends to contribute. Its objective is to help overcome this phase in the best possible way, without the need to resort to taking medicine or supplements. In each chapter you will find a simple explanation of why each principal symptom occurs, as well as diet programs and exercise that can contribute to facing them efficiently. Of course, the principal health problems associated with menopause are also included.

If you take the advice that you will read seriously and you make the necessary lifestyle changes, you will be able to go through this stage without too much stress and, most importantly, while maintaining enviable cardiovascular health and agile and strong bones.

To facilitate the diet programs that this book contains, in the last chapter you will find some guidelines that will help you organize yourself and plan your most appropriate diet.

Menopause, a Step Forward

Puberty, pregnancy, and menopause are the three great stages of transition that take place throughout the life of a woman. Each of them leads us to a new life cycle, and it is absolutely normal that during its course we experience great physical, emotional, and psychological changes.

Understanding why these changes—which we sometimes experience with certain fear and confusion—arise, can help us to better understand ourselves. But, above all, it will help us to accept our female condition with pride and gratefulness, without rejecting or being embarrassed by some of the often irritating consequences that these transition periods often entail.

Puberty: Hormonal Awakening

When a girl is born, she comes into the world with a generous amount of oocyte (or eggs), around 500,000. These sexual cells are accumulated in the ovaries but not in an isolated form; rather, each of them is surrounded by a layer of another type of cell forming what is known as "ovarian follicles." During childhood, the combination of ovules remains inactive until, at around eight years old, an endocrine gland located in the brain (the pineal gland) emits a signal that turns on the female reproduction system. Then puberty begins.

Puberty is a period of transition in which childhood is left behind and gives way to adolescence. You probably remember the rapid, spectacular changes—mostly physical—that you experienced as you transitioned out of childhood: you grew a lot, you started to develop breasts, you grew hair in your armpits and on your pubis . . . and one day you had your first period. The first period or "menarche" normally takes place between ten and sixteen years of age, and with it puberty comes to an end.

All the changes that are produced during this transition are directed by hormones. These chemical substances are generated in the endocrine glands and their principal function is to transmit information between different organs and systems of the body. The hypothalamus (structure located in the brain) is the "command center" and the first to act. The gonadotropin-releasing hormone (GnRH) sends the order to the hypophysis (gland close to the hypothalamus) to produce other hormones whose mission will be to direct other endocrine glands in the body, among which are the ovaries (also the testicles, the thyroid, and the adrenal glands).

The hormones secreted by the hypophysis (or pituitary gland) that head towards the ovaries are the gonadotropins (follicle-stimulating hormone, or FSH, and luteinizing hormone, or LH). Their function is to stimulate the ovaries (and also the testicles) so they begin to produce estrogen, progesterone, and testosterone. These sex hormones will be the protagonists of many of the changes that will mark our lives from this point on.

During puberty, estrogen is responsible for the development of secondary sexual characteristics. In other words, it's estrogen that orders the breasts to grow and the internal genitals (uterus and vagina) to mature. The first menstruation indicates that the levels of estrogen have already increased enough for the uninterrupted cyclical process to begin, the maturity of eggs that will try to be fertile throughout the entire fertile stage. Nevertheless, of the initial amount, only four hundred eggs mature enough and will be released during the menstrual cycle. The others will deteriorate little by little over time.

Progesterone appears later, when the ovaries have already started to function. Their function is to make the endometrium (the internal lining of the uterus) grow, and ultimately to prepare it to accommodate, protect, and nourish the fertilized egg, were it given the chance. When fertilization does not take place, progesterone and estrogen levels diminish, the lining dissolves, and menstruation takes place.

Adulthood: Relative Stability

We hardly realize we have left adolescence behind when we enter adulthood. In this stage, we have achieved our complete physical development and we live in a period of relative psychological and emotional stability. In any case, however stable your life may be, the new challenges that present themselves daily challenge you to never stop learning.

From the hormonal perspective, adulthood coincides with our reproductive years, which is characterized by the changes related to the menstrual cycle. This cyclical process begins the first day of the period, whose duration can be between two and seven days, and ends between twenty-three and twenty-five days later, depending on each woman's individual experience. The mission of this cycle is to prepare the body for eventual pregnancy (if it does not happen, the period arrives). The follicle-stimulating hormone (FSH) and the luteinizing hormone (LH) are secreted by the pituitary gland, and estrogen and progesterone are produced by the ovaries and intervene in its regulation.

During this stage, many women also experience motherhood. This phase includes pregnancy, giving birth, and nursing as well as other postnatal demands on the body. It is a period of intense physiological changes augmented by abrupt hormonal fluctuations. This period of transition especially affects the emotions. In fact, it is usual that the woman has conflicting emotions: on one side, pregnancy is reason for great happiness; on the other, the cause of many fears.

And Then . . . Menopause Arrives

One day, at around forty years old, our internal clock changes rhythms and ovarian senescence begins. From that moment on, just like in puberty, other hormonal changes take place that make way for many changes. From forty on, ovulation does not take place in an orderly way every month, and consequently menstrual cycles become irregular in intensity, duration, and frequency: some months the period arrives late, but others it arrives early, sometimes even multiple months can pass between periods. And, along with the menstrual irregularity, we begin to experience annoying symptoms that we didn't before. Yes, hot flashes, night sweats, insomnia, fatigue, mood changes . . . interrupt our lives without warning and, unless these changes are very severe, our periods continue like this until one day is the last time—in other words, one day the period will not return because we have arrived at menopause.

The premenopausal symptoms can appear up to ten years before the period ends completely. Nevertheless, before the initial signs of discomfort, many women are scared because they are not conscious of what is happening to them. This occurs because, even though we have all heard menopause talked about, what happens to us throughout its course has not always been explained to us well. To be well informed about what this life cycle involves is necessary in order to be prepared and to face it successfully. Recognizing the symptoms early on will allow you to be conscious of the fact that you are in the middle of a process of change, and that way you will be able to dedicate the time and care necessary to go through this stage in the best possible way.

Keep in mind that if we take advantage of this moment, in spite of the discomfort that adaptation to this new situation involves, menopause creates an opportunity for us to create a new, fuller, and gratifying life, in all aspects.

What Is Menopause? Definitions

People often tend to confuse the many terms used to refer to this stage of life. Because of this, before going on, it is important to clarify the meaning of the most relevant terms.

"Menopause" is the medical term that marks the date of the last menstruation in a woman's life. It is a natural physiological event that involves decreased production of the hormones that are generated in the ovaries, estrogen and progesterone. It takes place at around fifty years of age (between forty-five and fifty-five) and is accompanied by the loss of the ability to reproduce. If this process takes place in a natural way, the woman will not know if a period is the last one until twelve months have passed. Because of this, a woman can only be sure that she has passed through menopause after the fact, once a year has passed since the final period.

The period disappears suddenly one day in few cases. Except 10 percent of women who have their last period overnight with nothing more, the majority of us pass through a transition preceding the date of menopause.

This period beforehand lasts between eight and ten years, and during its course the quantity of said hormones gradually diminishes. This period of transition is what is known as "perimenopause," which refers to approximately one year after menopause. While it occurs we lose ovarian follicles at an accelerated rate, until they finally run out. Some experts also use the term "perimenopause" to name the years that precede menopause, where a series of varied low-intensity changes are produced. For example, menstrual cycles tend to be regular, but it is already possible to experience the occasional hot flash. However, the WHO (World Health Organization) recommends that the word "perimenopause" be used to refer to the woman's entire fertile period until the moment of menopause.

Meanwhile, postmenopause begins after menopause and lasts approximately eight or ten years. In this stage many symptoms of perimenopause diminish in intensity. In exchange, due to various factors, in addition to the diminishment of estrogen levels, a higher risk of illnesses like osteoporosis and cardiovascular problems arises.

The term "menopause" is often used to refer to the entire transitional spectrum, including perimenopause and postmenopause. The actual stage of menopause occurs between perimenopause and postmenopause. Its duration can be between five and fifteen years. "Climacteric" is another term that may be used to describe the entire spectrum: perimenopause, menopause, and postmenopause. So, even though menopause is technically only one phase, we often use the term to talk about the entire transitional period, from initial imbalances until our bodies finally adapt to the new physiological situation.

Phases of Menopause

* **Perimenopause** is the stage that precedes menopause and ends one year after the last period. It can last months, although most typically it lasts eight to ten years. It tends to be accompanied by irregular menstrual cycles.

* **Menopause** itself refers to the date in which the last definitive period takes place. It is understood that twelve months must have passed since menstruation to be sure that it has taken place.

* **Postmenopause** is the stage that includes approximately the ten years following the last period. The diminishment of estrogen and progesterone in this period provokes the appearance of some health problems in a high percentage of cases, although not always with the same intensity.

Premature Menopause

Menopause can happen naturally, prematurely, or artificially. In approximately 90 percent of women who have at least one ovary, menopause happens naturally. The average age in which this phenomenon takes place is fifty years old, ranging between forty-five and fifty-five years. In the case of natural menopause, it presents itself little by little, and the duration of the perimenopause phase tends to last between eight and ten years, although sometimes it can last up to fifteen years.

Premature menopause is that which presents itself before forty years of age as a consequence of ovarian failure. It can be due to various causes, including genetic predisposition and certain immune disorders that produce antibodies that affect the ovaries and other organs.

Smoking or other types of chronic stress (for example, excessive physical exercise) are also associated with premature menopause. In this case, perimenopause tends to last longer than usual, from one to three years, which means more dramatic hormonal changes, more intense discomfort, and greater risk of developing osteoporosis during postmenopause. Because of this, it can be helpful to use hormone replacement therapy during the period of adaptation in cases of premature menopause.

Lastly, artificial menopause is that which originates as a result of surgical interventions in which, for different reasons, the ovaries are removed. It can also be induced by radiotherapy or chemotherapy, or because of taking certain medicines that provoke the situation. Since menopause occurs all of a sudden, the body does not have time to adapt to the hormonal drop slowly. Most of the time, a woman in this situation should resort to hormone replacement therapy, since symptoms will be very unpleasant and debilitating.

Hot Flashes and Much More

Although menopause is not an illness, the hormonal fluctuation that it produces can provoke the appearance of a wide variety of physical, emotional, and psychological symptoms. Hot flashes are among the most frequent of these symptoms that appear early. Others that also interrupt life in this stage are those that have to do with the emotional sphere, like irritability, anxiety, confusion, mood changes, or even depression. Because of this, during this period of transition you may get irritated easily or overreact to things that you managed before without difficulty. It is also likely that, sometimes, you feel confused and insecure in situations that did not provoke any discomfort previously.

Other changes that can form part of the menopause line-up are fatigue and insomnia, as well as migraines, which can present themselves very intensely, even without having previously experienced them.

Some women pass through perimenopause with little discomfort, but the truth is that in our society there is a large number of us who do suffer through it. But, even if your symptoms are more intense, do not think they will remain with you for the rest of your life. In a natural transition, perimenopause lasts five to ten years. In the beginning, symptoms appear punctually; with the course of time, it gradually spreads out, and as the date of menopause gets closer, they reach their height. However, during postmenopause they diminish to reestablish new hormonal balance within the new rhythm to which the body is adapting. So, don't worry because this discomfort will pass and disappear in the same way it appeared.

The problem comes because, aside from these symptoms produced by hormonal fluctuations, the decrease of estrogen is also associated with other changes that aren't so fleeting. These are disorders that, in addition to depending on hormonal levels, are also bound to the process of aging, which contains greater wear and tear and deterioration of health in general. In fact, it is not always possible to distinguish the changes that originate because of menopause from those related to age. So, for example, it is possible that you start to notice discomfort that derives from atrophy of the urogenital epithelium or that you perceive the beginning of a change in your skin's appearance. Another health problem that can occur in postmenopause is osteoporosis. Postmenopause also sparks the risk of cardiovascular illness, although, not long ago drop in estrogen was blamed, and the actual cause is no longer clear.

Everything Is Because of Hormonal Revolution

When the definite cease of the period takes place, the amount of estrogen and progesterone is really very low. But, in the years before this moment, the levels of these hormones fluctuate so much that there are even periods of time in which estrogen levels are much higher than normal (situation of estrogen dominance). Meanwhile, levels of follicle stimulating hormones and luteinizing hormones that the hypophysis secretes also become irregular. So, the cause of climacteric symptoms does not always manifest in a deficit of estrogen, as is often said, rather in the hormonal revolution that takes place during the perimenopausal transition.

Beginning with menopause, the amounts of hypophysis hormones are much higher than normal and they remain that way afterwards. On the other hand, from this moment on the levels of estrogen and progesterone will remain diminished.

Ovaries Do Not Stop Working

Although the belief is common that beginning in menopause the ovaries wear out and stop working, this is not quite the case. Menopause is an absolutely normal event and it is programmed to take place. Because of this, it is an error to refer to it as a "an ovarian error" or "an ovarian insufficiency." What happens to these glands is that they change gears and become slower, just as nature had planned.

Keep in mind that, in contrast to what happens during our fertile years, when we enter maturity, we no longer need high levels of sex hormones to be able to reproduce. However, the body will continue secreting them, although in lesser quantities, so that they can accomplish tasks other than reproduction. No wonder almost all of the organs and tissues in our body present receptors for estrogen. Additionally, apart from the ovaries, other centers capable of producing estrogen (for example fat tissue) exist for when it is necessary.

Take Care of Yourself and You Will Have Minimal Discomfort

If you take care of your physical and psychological health your body will be capable of facing all the hormonal challenges that it is presented with, now and for the rest of your life. Additionally, you will probably have little discomfort during the perimenopause transition and you will be able to begin your second path of life with energy and good health.

Nowadays it is common to have a difficult menopause due to the lifestyle that we tend to lead. In our society it is not unusual to find women who follow disorderly and unbalanced diets; or who do not move enough because they are sedentary; or who smoke and drink too much alcohol. It is also common that we are overcome by stress, whether we pressure ourselves to achieve unrealistic domestic or work-related goals, or for any other reason. The case is that we live with stress and hurrying every day and they do not allow us to be able to have a moment alone with ourselves. Of course this lifestyle does not help us at all. In fact, it is seriously harmful to our health, especially in perimenopause, a time in which what we most need is harmony and tranquility to be able to reestablish our hormonal balance in a natural way.

Menopause is a good time to reflect and take a look at your life. If you feel good and satisfied with it, well, how wonderful! Keep it up. But, if you don't feel well physically, or you don't like what you have achieved up to this point and you feel frustrated, or you simply don't know what direction to head, now is the moment to get to work and start to trust yourself. Address everything that robs you of energy or that doesn't make you feel good, and of course, change the unhealthy habits that deteriorate your health.

Contemplate all aspects of your life and shape your new life plan with the objective to improve and strengthen it. The advice you will find throughout this book will help you to create conditions so that you can live the second stage of your life with more health, happiness, and fullness.

But, before delving into what you can do to improve your health and alleviate each symptom that the hormonal confusion can cause throughout menopause, let's see what hormone replacement therapy consists of, its pros and cons. It is important that you know why so many health professionals still use and advise the use of these treatments, despite the known harm that this type of treatment can cause to a woman's health.

Hormone Replacement Therapy

Hormone replacement therapy (HRT) consists of administering hormones—estrogen and progestogen—to replace those that the ovaries no longer produce, in order to avoid symptoms. Many doctors recommend this therapy to relieve some of the most common symptoms of perimenopause and also to prevent osteoporosis in the long-term. Generally the treatment is comprised of just estrogen, a combination of estrogen and progesterone, or estrogen and progestin, which is a synthetic hormone with similar effects to those of progesterone.

For example, estrogen and progestin are prescribed to women whose reproductive system remains intact, because the treatment with only estrogen is associated with an increased risk of endometrial cancer. However, studies show that the combination of hormones mentioned doesn't necessarily have this effect.

But, although HRT provides some short term benefits, like relief from hot flashes and discomfort from urogenital atrophy as well as an increase in bone mineral density, it is not free of very significant risks. For example, it is proven that HRT increases the risk for certain types of cancer. In fact, it is the pharmaceutical treatment that has generated the most investigation and controversy in the past decades.

In the face of the unfavorable results of many of the studies that have been completed to evaluate its risks and benefits, the United States Food and Drug Administration (FDA) currently advises the use of HRT for the shortest amount of time possible and in the lowest dose possible to control the symptoms of menopause. Likewise, the Spanish Agency of Medicine (*Agencia Española del Medicamento*), like other international agencies, considers the use of HRT to be unjustifiable in women with light symptoms.

Risks of Hormone Replacement Therapy

Until recently, the use of HRT was also recommended for the prevention of cardiovascular illness, since it was believed that this treatment protected women in this area. However, nowadays it is known that, not only does it not protect, rather it increases the chance of brain damage. Large-scale studies have shown that HRT increases the risk of cardiovascular illness, venous thrombosis (above all in women who smoke), and brain damage. For example, one of the studies that has most thoroughly investigated this topic is the *Heart and Estrogen/Progestin Replacement Study* (HERS), in which over almost seven years they observed 2,763 postmenopausal North American women with histories of heart disease. The results proved that those who were treated with HRT did not have lower cardiovascular risks. However, other data indicated an increase in said risk in postmenopausal women who did not have a history of coronary disease, but who were treated with HRT.

With respect to the risk of developing some types of cancer, studies exist principally for breast, endometrial, and ovarian cancers. For breast cancer, there is no doubt: HRT increases the risk. Results of different studies have shown this increased risk, and additionally it has been proven that the risk is proportional with the duration of the treatment. In cases of endometrial cancer, it is shown that the administration of estrogen in an isolated form increases the risk. And, with regards to ovarian cancer, although the most recent studies have been unable to show significant data, observations have been made in studies that show a higher rate of this type of cancer in women with long-term use of HRT (over ten years).

Another demonstrated effect of HRT is the increase in risk of gallstones. And, as if all of this weren't enough, although it is proven that synthetic estrogen increases bone mineral density, a study exists in which ten years after having suspended the hormonal treatment, both bone density and risk of fracture were similar to those of women who had never been treated with replacement hormones.

Other Side Effects and Risks

Some of the most common side effects that HRT can also produce are: headache, stomachache, stomach distension, diarrhea, increase in appetite and weight gain, anxiety, mood swings, spots on the skin, acne, retention of liquids, changes in menstrual flow, mammary gland sensitivity, and chest growth. These changes vary depending on the form in which the hormones are administered.

What's more, HRT is not recommended as a definitive treatment in cases of undiagnosed vaginal bleeding, liver disease, pregnancy, arterial coronary disease, venous thrombosis, and if there are signs of endometrial cancer. It is also not recommended, unless it offers greater benefit than risk, in cases of migraines, patients with histories of ovarian or breast cancer, risk of gallstones, atypical ductal hyperplasia in the breast (a risk factor for breast cancer), or liver disease. Women who smoke should also not use HRT.

Of course, due to all that is involved in HRT, this treatment should only be used in exceptional cases and under strict medical supervision.

Considering Pharmaceuticals

In our society, around 80 percent of perimenopausal women have symptoms that are intense and bothersome enough to have to seek out some resource that can relieve them. But, if this is your case, first of all do not forget that menopause is not an illness and that its symptoms will taper off after a few years.

Remember that our body, if we take care of it and respect it, is prepared with everything it needs to face this period of change and reestablish its hormonal equilibrium without the need to turn to pharmaceuticals.

Clearly, good medical advice is always recommended, which, if necessary, will help you weigh the pros and cons of taking a therapeutic drug. But don't take the first one you see right away due to pressure from the media or some health professionals who are in favor of HRT. Before deciding to take hormones, reflect on what is happening to you and weigh whether the risks involved in this treatment are worth the few benefits it contributes. Ask your doctor for advice and express all your doubts and fears. Ask him or her for the recommendation he or she sees most fit for you, why he or she sees it that way, and most importantly, ask to have your symptoms and possible side-effects evaluated. And, when it comes time to decide, it should be clear that the decision is only yours.

It is also important that before taking a hormonal treatment to relieve discomfort, which satisfies the commercial interest of pharmaceutical companies, that you search for more options. In many cases, where there is a little discomfort and no other health problems, it is enough to adopt a healthy lifestyle that includes healthy and balanced eating, regular physical exercise, and the practice of a relaxation technique (to connect with your inner-self). It is also very helpful and comforting to attend to our needs regarding our inner growth. In fact, menopause is a great moment for our evolution. But, if it is not enough to relieve your symptoms, you can also resort to a good therapist who can direct you to other alternative therapies (like herbal medicine, homeopathy, or acupuncture, among others) that can be just as efficient as HRT but are much more respectful of your feminine condition.

Hot Flashes, Those Heat Waves

The vasomotor symptoms, or hot flashes as they are commonly known, are the most common symptom that we endure throughout perimenopause. It is calculated that they affect 80 percent of western women in this stage and, although they are not dangerous, they can be quite bothersome. Every woman experiences them in a different way. Because of their varied presentation and frequency, it is difficult to define them in exact terms. So, as much as hot flashes are described to you, you won't know what they are like until you experience the first one.

A hot flash begins with a sudden wave of intense heat in the upper part of the chest and in the face that later flows throughout the entire body. It frequently produces sweat and palpitations and the skin turns red. Sometimes it also is accompanied by a tingling sensation in the hands, weakness, and even dizziness, and it is common to experience cold and chills after the heat. This vasomotor instability lasts approximately three to six minutes, although it can also be very mild and last just a few seconds. Similarly, some women only experience one a month, while others have one every half hour.

The majority of women in perimenopause have hot flashes sporadically and of moderate intensity. However, between 10 and 15 percent of perimenopausal women present them very frequently and severely, according to statistics. When they are very intense they can interfere with rest to the point that they prevent sleep completely. This situation is very severe because the women can end up suffering depression due to lack of sleep.

What Are Palpitations?

Palpitations are rapid heartbeats that come about unexpectedly. They can appear at any hour of the day but are more frequent at night.

When cardiac rhythm accelerates without warning, it is normal to be alarmed as it is a symptom associated with cardiovascular disease. However, palpitations that are accompanied by hot flashes are rarely dangerous. Normally they are related to a hormonal imbalance involved in perimenopause, although sometimes they can also be influenced by the anxiety that this life stage produces in us.

In any case, consult your doctor if they persist.

Hot flashes do not appear in our lives all of a sudden, but rather they come on little by little, according to what we go through in perimenopause. Forty-one percent of women with a history of twenty-nine or more years of regular cycles experience them sporadically. But, while they create a lack of control of estrogen levels, they increase in frequency and intensity until they reach their peak at the end of menstruation.

Because of this, having occasional hot flashes in your forties can be the first sign that menopause is getting nearer.

Beginning on the date of menopause, vasomotor symptoms persist for a period of two to three years. Afterwards, they diminish progressively until they disappear completely (in some cases they could last longer).

Why Do They Happen?

Many hypotheses exist with regard to the cause (or causes) of hot flashes. But an exact scientific reason for why they exist is still unknown. What does seem to be confirmed is their relation to hormonal changes that are produced during this transition period.

On the other hand, their characteristics seem to correspond to a change in the control of temperature regulation, located in the hypothalamus. It is suspected that one factor that could activate the mechanism is the loss of heat, which is accompanied by dilation of the blood vessels in the skin of the head and neck. This would provoke the flow of more blood to this zone, which would produce a great sensation of heat and sweat. Later, the heat conservation mechanism would be stimulated with vasoconstriction and chills.

What Can Relieve Them?

At least initially, hot flashes are harmless and do not require treatment. Because of this, if you are one of women who have them mildly or moderately, you will probably be able to avoid them becoming a problem with the following methods.

To begin, it is convenient to know that, although they tend to come about spontaneously, factors exist that influence their intensity and duration. For example, tobacco and alcoholic beverages do not only bring them about, but they can also strengthen them. Nervousness, anxiety, and emotional or physical stress also promote them. A sedentary lifestyle, as well as elevated temperatures in the summer, can accentuate them.

Revise Your Diet

Among factors that influence the frequency and severity of vasomotor symptoms is diet. A healthy and balanced diet is always a fundamental pillar to promote health and prevent the development of countless problems. But, this is most important from forty years on, when we are faced with overcoming challenges that we will surely encounter.

In the last chapter of this book you will find more information about a diet that will be most convenient for you in your second life cycle. For now, in this section you have the advice on diets that work best and worst for managing hot flashes.

Light, Mild Meals

It is traditional to believe that hot or spicy dishes or dishes with lots of seasoning can trigger vasomotor symptoms. This assumption is not accompanied by enough scientific evidence to be able to affirm that it is true. However, it is true that many women are able to alleviate this discomfort by eliminating this type of dish from their diet. Therefore, although this preventative recommendation does not have scientific basis, you do not lose anything by trying it to see if light and mild dishes sit better with you during this climacteric transition.

What is confirmed is that caffeine, alcoholic beverages, and smoking are factors that worsen both the intensity and the frequency of hot flashes.

The Coffee Dilemma

Coffee owes its stimulating effect to caffeine, a substance from the group of xanthines that also is found in tea, chocolate, and cola drinks. There is nothing that stimulates you more than having a cup of coffee in the first hour of the day. However, drinking it in excess is considered counterproductive for your health.

Now, although its abuse is not recommended, the number of studies that demonstrate the beneficial effects of this drink is increasing. For example, some experts have demonstrated that strong black coffee, contributes to better blood circulation, which assists cardiovascular health. Similarly, studies exist that show that it keeps brain functions from slowing down from cognitive deterioration. So, moderate consumption of coffee can be a good idea for health.

In any case, it's not all good news. A survey from the Mayo Clinic taken by more than 1,800 menopausal women that was published in the magazine *Menopause*, affirms that drinking coffee or other caffeinated beverages triggers hot flashes and night sweats, although it increases mood, concentration, and memory. At present, this study is the best study done on effects of caffeine on the symptoms of menopause. Although its findings are preliminary, the conclusion is clear: if your vasomotor symptoms do not change your life too much, you can drink between two and three cups of coffee a day without a problem. But, if you experience very bothersome hot flashes, it would be good for you to eliminate this drink (as well as tea and sodas), at least until the symptoms diminish.

Light, Lowfat Diet

The North American Menopause Society (NAMS) affirms that night sweats are associated with elevated levels of cholesterol in the blood, So, it benefits you to follow a light diet that is low in saturated and trans fats as well as low in refined sugars (this will not only help improve hot flashes, but also many other health problems).

Some studies have found that women who follow a diet similar to that of the Mediterranean are less likely to suffer vasomotor symptoms. The basic foods of this type of diet (and that offer the most benefits) are fresh fruit and vegetables, whole-grains, legumes, nuts, fish, and extra virgin olive oil. It also includes white meats, like fish and rabbit, and red meat in small quantities. Therefore, pre-cooked or industrially processed foods don't have a place. So, it could be said that the Mediterranean diet is characterized for being light and rich in vegetables full of vitamins, minerals, fiber, and many other phytonutrients beneficial for good health. It also has the distinctive feature of contributing a good quantity of unsaturated fats, while supplying very few saturated or trans fats, sugars, and refined flours.

This type of diet, in addition to reducing hot flashes, also contributes to preventing cardiovascular illness, cognitive impairment (it diminishes the risk of suffering from dementia), certain types of cancer (like breast or colon cancers), and obesity, among other benefits. Because of this, whether or not you present vasomotor symptoms, to overcome the symptoms of menopause with success, it would do you well to modify your diet to follow a similar model to the Mediterranean diet.

Avoid Weight Gain

Weight gain, or worse yet, obesity, in addition to increasing the risk of developing many illnesses, also predisposes you for more frequent and intense hot flashes.

In *The Women's Health Initiative Dietary Modification Trial* of 17,473 postmenopausal women between the ages of fifty and seventy-nine, they studied the effect of following a diet low in fat and high in vegetables (like the aforementioned diet) and weight loss in perimenopausal symptoms (none of the included women took HRT).

The investigators observed that women who followed this type of diet presented fewer symptoms, in comparison with the control group. In addition, they proved that if they lost weight (at least 10 percent of their body weight), their symptoms diminished, unlike those who didn't lose weight. So, the conclusion they reached from this study was that weight loss due to a diet low in fat and high in fruits, vegetables, and whole grains contributes to reducing menopausal symptoms, especially hot flashes and night sweats.

Taking Care with Soy

Nowadays the use of various plants, foods, and dietary supplements to reduce the vasomotor symptoms of menopause has become more common. But be careful, because some of these substances have not yet been studied well in rigorous clinical trials, because of which, unfortunately, it is not completely proven that they do not have negative effects.

One of the most famous and recognized fuels of this type is soy. Surely you have heard or read in magazines, books, newspapers, television, etc., that you should have more soy (or one of its derivatives) to forget about symptoms of menopause. It could even be that someone you trust recommended it to you. The point is that this legume is omnipresent in all markets in our lives. You can buy soy drinks (incorrectly called "soy milk"), tofu, miso, tempeh, tamari (soy sauce), soy yogurt . . . or, if you prefer, you can take it in capsules or tablets.

True, the enormous interest that this legume solicits is due to its content in isoflavones. Because of this it is considered a beneficial fuel for good health and a useful natural alternative in the treatment of symptoms associated with menopause. However, although it has been used to reduce these symptoms for a few decades, not too much reliable data is available that proves that soy really helps control them.

Phytoestrogens

Isoflavones are a type of phytoestrogen. These compounds are not only found in soy, but also form part of many foods of plant origin like whole grains, legumes, leafy vegetables, and fruits. More than 4,000 have been described and grouped into four families: lignans, coumestans, isoflavones, and resorcylic acid lactones, although these last ones are less relevant in human nutrition.

All phytoestrogens identified have a common molecular self with a chemical structure very similar to that of estrogen, natural (17 beta-estradiol) as well as synthetic. For this reason, these compounds possess weak estrogen activity, which sparks their interest in relation to symptoms of menopause.

* The Isoflavones of Soy

Isoflavones constitute the most numerous and studied family of phytoestrogens. These compounds are found in all legumes, although the most abundant source is the soy seed and some of its derivatives. According to the conclusions of epidemiological studies done a few years ago, a diet rich in isoflavones reduces the incidence of menopausal symptoms, especially hot flashes. These same studies also assured that these substances diminished the risk of cardiovascular illness and improved osteoporosis, symptoms also associated with menopause. For this reason, when faced with the logical fear involved in using HRT, supplements with a high percentage of isoflavones constitute the most frequently used alternative treatment.

* All That Glitters Is Not Gold

However, while studies exist ensuring that soy has beneficial properties, some experts also support other studies that have put many of the benefits associated with this legume to question. Because of this, although the food industry does not tire of promoting its virtues (in fact, soy is becoming present in a wider and wider range of products) it is very difficult to have a true opinion about its properties.

With regard to supplements of isoflavones, studies also exist with contradictory results that indicate either that they are not efficient or even that they can be counterproductive for a woman's health. For example, according to conclusions of a study published by the University of Miami in *Archives of Internal Medicine* in 2011, the supplements of isoflavones of soy are not effective in preventing hot flashes, vaginal dryness, disruption of sleep, or bone loss in the first five years of menopause.

25

Another study published in the *Journal of the National Cancer Institute* (JNCI) in 2014 concluded that the administration of soy supplements alter the expression of genes associated with breast cancer, and said investigation consequently planted the possibility that soy could exert a stimulating effect on breast cancer in a subset of women. In fact, women with histories of breast cancer are advised against the use of these supplements because some pre-clinical studies have already showed that a higher risk could exist when using high doses of phytoestrogens during prolonged periods of time. The daily dose of isoflavones that is currently used is between 40 and 80 mg/day with a minimum of 15 mg of Genistein, which has no known side-effects. However, more studies are still necessary to guarantee their long-term safety, since the effects of high doses of isoflavones administered in an isolated form are still relatively unknown. Before taking this type of product we should reflect on whether we really need them or if we can do without them. It is also necessary to seek out a good professional's assessment. And, of course, the most important is that we follow our common sense and intuition.

Flax Seeds

Another highly recommended food to soothe vasomotor symptoms is flax seeds. Flax contains lignans, which are another type of phytoestrogen. Because of this it was thought that, like soy, taking a daily serving of 40 grams of these ground seeds would help reduce hot flashes. In fact, preliminary studies carried out in 2007 in the United States suggested that flax seeds had this effect. However, a more recent investigation from the Mayo Clinic concluded that the flax seed does not offer advantages to improve hot flashes among postmenopausal women.

This being said, although flax seeds do not help to alleviate vasomotor symptoms, they do offer other benefits. The most prominent characteristic of flax seeds is the ability to combat constipation due to their high fiber content. They also have properties that are good for the heart because of their content of unsaturated fatty-acids and omega 3. And, although more evidence is still required, flax seeds are also attributed protective properties against certain types of cancer. Now, while this effect is probably due to its content of lignans, as long as there is no information regarding the way they work (for or against tumor growth), the most prudent action to take in case of suffering a hormone-dependent tumor (like breast cancer, or endometrial cancer) is to avoid excess.

Exercise More

In addition to eating healthily and lightly, staying active is also fundamental to control vasomotor symptoms. Although it has not been proven that exercise improves these symptoms, it is a reality that women who practice some physical activity in a moderate and regular fashion suffer fewer hot flashes. Additionally, what we do know with certainty is that a sedentary lifestyle serves as a trigger for this particular symptom.

On the other hand, strengthening the circulatory system can also contribute to less intense vasomotor instability with less frequency. Daily massages, saunas, or showers alternating cold and hot water strengthen the circulatory system and get it in shape, while making it more resistant to disorder.

Learn to Relax

Breathing techniques and muscular relaxation exercises tend to be used to control stress and have also been shown to be options capable of diminishing the intensity of hot flashes up to 40 percent, according to clinical studies. Not in vain, nervousness and anxiety aggravate vasomotor instability.

So, whether or not you are stressed, you should include the practice of one of these methods in your daily routine, because not only will it help you reduce hot flashes, but it will also improve your quality of life in general. For example, a very simple breathing technique that you can do at any moment of the day is rhythmic breathing. To practice, you simply must be sitting in a calm place and start to breathe slowly, deeply, and in a controlled manner. Fifteen minutes, twice a day, is enough to notice improvement.

Similarly, it has been proven that meditation techniques are also very effective to diminish the vasomotor symptoms of perimenopause, as well as yoga and tai chi.

Stay Away from Hot Environments

High temperatures favor hot flashes. On the other hand, these symptoms are much less frequent, shorter, and less intense in cold climates. Therefore, something as simple as avoiding hot environments and maintaining a fresher temperature wherever you find yourself will contribute to more sporadic hot flashes. And, when they present themselves, they will do so in a much softer and manageable way.

It would be ideal to maintain a constant temperature in your house of between 68 and 69.8 degrees Fahrenheit and that, to the extent possible, you try to avoid drastic and sudden changes in temperature. To better control heat it will also be useful to dress in light, loose-fitting clothing and in layers that you can take off or put on depending on what your body needs. Always carrying a fan in your bag is also an invaluable resource.

Alternative Therapies Also Help

If you integrate the practices that you just read about into your routine, hot flashes will probably not be a problem for you. But, if even with these suggestions you are unable to reduce them, keep in mind that some types of alternate therapies exist that can also be helpful, like cognitive behavioral therapy or herbal medicine. Really, some women have hot flashes so intense that they reduce their quality of life. Others, although they don't have them as severely, live in true desperation due to how uncomfortable and exasperating they can be.

Behavior Modification

Cognitive behavioral therapy is a very effective technique to control the vasomotor symptoms of perimenopause with the distinctive feature that it is a safe alternative lacking side-effects. It also offers additional benefits, like improving mood, sleep, and quality of life in general.

With this type of therapy you learn to face the perimenopausal transition with a healthier and more positive attitude. It focuses on modifying the negative beliefs you may have about menopause and the perception and interpretation of hot flashes. Because of this, although you continue having them, you hardly feel them and you have more faith in your ability to endure them.

Homeopathic Medicine

Another alternative treatment that can help you manage vasomotor symptoms is homeopathic medicine with the use of plants such as black cohosh, angelica sinensis (also known as dong quai, or "female ginseng"), red clover, or chaste tree. Now, since these plants contain phytoestrogen, you should not take them without previously consulting a good specialist, especially if you present a negative reaction to estrogen.

Keep in mind that they can have different effects, not only with regards to the dosage used, but also your hormonal status when you take them. Additionally, it has still not been confirmed that these plants are completely safe, in fact, some of them present side-effects that should be kept in mind.

Other options to soothe hot flashes, as well as other symptoms of menopause, are homeopathic medicine, acupuncture, and hypnosis.

Hormonal Treatment: Only in Special Cases

In cases of premature menopause or ovarian insufficiency induced by chemotherapy or surgical menopause, HRT is considered the most adequate treatment to alleviate hot flashes (estrogen diminishes hot flashes between 80 and 90 percent). These situations involve a very sudden hormonal change, with which the produced symptoms are very severe and unpleasant.

Now, in the case of natural menopause with light or moderate symptoms, it is not worth using this treatment and running the risks that it involves. In fact, in this situation its use is not advised. Remember that the techniques related to lifestyle and behavior also have demonstrated their effectiveness in diminishing the malaise associated with hot flashes.

Insomnia and How to Sleep Deeply Through the Night

A good night's rest is fundamental to feeling good in all aspects. Sleep is an active physiological state; during its course metabolic and hormonal changes take place that stimulate rest and recuperation of the brain and nervous system. During sleep, brain relaxation enables thought and intellectual activity, achieves the replacement of energy, and contributes to preserving memory and to restoring the immune system.

This is why sleep is basic for the body and mind to be able to function at 100 percent during the next day. Contrarily, when we sleep poorly or not at all, our health deteriorates: we are constantly drowsy, we feel tired, we make a mess of things, and we get irritated. And, if insomnia continues, we also become highly susceptible to depression. During the perimenopausal transition, difficulty falling asleep and waking up frequently are the order of the day.

For a while now, women as well as doctors related insomnia with hot flashes, although said association was never too clear. However, now this relationship has been confirmed thanks to a study carried out by University of Stanford (USA) and published in the magazine *Archives of Internal Medicine*, in which it was proven that chronic insomnia really increases dramatically among women who suffer from severe hot flashes. In fact, this disruption is especially serious in the case of surgical menopause, in which vasomotor symptoms are very strong in intensity.

Insomnia and Night Sweats

Hot flashes also are produced during the night (night sweats), with the defining characteristic that, when they appear while we sleep, they interrupt and wake us up hot, soaked in sweat, and many times with palpitations. If hot flashes are frequent, constant interruptions of sleep make it more difficult to return to sleep. The result is that many menopausal women cannot sleep, and when they do, they hardly get any rest.

Insomnia opens the door to other problems, for example, lack of energy or difficulty concentrating. But the worst is that of the 80 percent of women who suffer hot flashes, an estimated 15 percent experience a depressive state of mood. In fact, the more severe the hot flashes, the higher risk of suffering from depression.

Sleeping Pills Are Not the Answer

If insomnia is your problem, it is understandable that after spending restless nights you are tempted to take some sort of medicine to help you sleep. However, this is not the solution. It is true that in the case of sporadic insomnia due to jet lag or another isolated stressful situation (a move, a separation, etc.), taking pharmaceuticals to sleep can help you rest. But, when you suffer chronic insomnia as a consequence of night sweats, it is not advisable.

Keep in mind that these medicines create addiction, present side-effects (dizziness, facial swelling, headache, fatigue . . .) and additionally, they lose effectiveness, because you constantly need a higher dosage to achieve the same effect. Also, since they do not treat the cause of the insomnia, they do not resolve it. This creates a vicious cycle after beginning to use them that is hard to break. In fact, many experts advise against sleeping pills and only recommend their use as a last resort, over a short amount of time, and always under a medical prescription.

Now, what you can do to improve your night's rest is to revise and correct, if necessary, your life habits, especially schedules, exercise routine, and diet. Of course, the advice you have seen to alleviate hot flashes is also beneficial to you, because, if you manage to reduce your vasomotor symptoms, it is very likely that you will be able to sleep better.

Herbal Medicine Offers Natural Help

Medicinal plants sedate and calm nerves and relax muscles, which helps reconcile sleep and improve its quality. Some of the most common, effective, and safe (for lack of side-effects) herbal medicines of this type are lime blossom, passionflower, orange blossom, valerian, and hop.

The First Step to Deep Sleep: Schedule

If you keep in mind that a night's rest is one of the keys to vitality, creativity, or the motivation that you will have the next day, it is worth putting in the work to try to sleep better.

To start with, take care of your sleep routines. Begin by establishing a set time to go to sleep and wake up every day, and follow it. The brain has its own internal clock that regulates daily rhythms of the body with regards to the sleep-wakefulness cycle, because of which the hour of day can determine whether or not you are sleepy.

Following a routine every night before going to bed serves to make your brain understand that the time to rest is approaching. Dimming the brightness of the lights, putting on your pajamas, brushing your teeth, etc., are all small gestures that suggest that the end of the day has arrived. Similarly, reading a few pages of a light book, listening to soft music, relaxing herbal teas, etc. help to calm you and to be better prepared to go to sleep. And, of course, try to put work, family, or personal problems aside, since worrying functions as a powerful interrupter of sleep.

A favorable environment to rest is also fundamental; your room should be dark, without noise, with good ventilation, and at a comfortable temperature between 64 and 68 degrees Fahrenheit (an excess of cold or heat alters rest).

The Second Step: A Light and Relaxing Dinner

Apart from night sweats, other factors can cause you to not sleep or to sleep poorly. Some are obvious and we are familiar with them, like stress, disappointments, changes in work shifts, etc. But others also exist that are not always associated with insomnia, like diet. That being said, many times a balanced diet that is light and rich in relaxing properties help make a night's rest much better.

Foods That Don't Let You Sleep

All foods that compose a day's dinner influence sleep. For example, if your dinner is too copious or is high in saturated fat (meat fat, cold cuts, cheeses, pre-cooked dishes, sauces, fried food, etc.), or contains an excessive quantity of protein, you probably will have a long and heavy digestion process that will make falling asleep more difficult. Additionally, eating this sort of heavy dinner can cause an excess of digestive activity that can bring on heartburn. Because it is the last ingestion of the day, the excess energy will also make you gain weight. Keep in mind that while you sleep, you burn fewer calories than when you are active, and the body stores any extra energy in the form of fat.

It is also more difficult to get to sleep after a spicy or very seasoned dinner. Many spices, especially spicy ones, accelerate the metabolism and increase body temperature. In addition, it appears that in many women they cause hot flashes, which makes it clear that they are not effective in trying to solve the problem of insomnia. In their place try to use aromatic herbs with digestive or carminative features like fennel, oregano, or cumin. These condiments assist the digestive process and help avoid gas, which, in an indirect way, can contribute to improving your night's rest.

Foods that cause gas like legumes, vegetables from the cabbage family, or raw onion are also inadequate for dinner. There is no doubt that these foods are very healthy and of course your diet should not be missing them. But, despite their many benefits, they present the inconvenience that they create gas and cause abdominal bloating, which can make digestion and even getting to sleep more difficult. Because of this, it is preferable that you eat this sort of food at the midday meal.

Of course it also does not do you any good to drink alcoholic beverages nor stimulants like coffee. Alcohol makes you fall asleep faster, but it causes you to have a less still sleep from which you wake up often. Additionally, it provokes headaches and intensifies hot flashes.

With regards to coffee, you should not drink it more than six hours before going to bed. You know that this drink contains caffeine and that this substance activates you in such a way that it can prevent you from falling sleep. In addition to coffee, do not forget that tea, chocolate, and cola sodas also have caffeine, so they are also unadvisable at night.

Early Dinner

To be able to have a good, restorative sleep it is fundamental that you go to bed with digestion complete. Because of this it does you well to have dinner early and to let at least two hours pass before going to sleep. If you delay the hour of the last meal of the day, you will be forced to go straight to bed, in the middle of the digestive process, and this will interfere with your rest.

Sleep Facilitators

A complete, but light, dinner facilitates digestion and will not provoke problems when it is time to rest. You have already seen that abundant dinners rich in proteins and saturated fats make getting to sleep more difficult. Now, eating a light dinner does not necessarily mean that you only eat a little or eat just a piece of fruit or a yogurt. The ideal is to eat a salad or another plate of simply cooked vegetables first, and white fish, chicken, turkey, or an egg with a light dressing, and a piece of fruit or a nonfat yogurt for dessert.

The fact that you should avoid an excess of protein at dinner time does not take away the fact that you need to include an adequate portion of protein at dinner time. You already know that too much of this nutrient complicates digestion, but in the right quantity it will give you the essential amino acids your body needs for the formation and reparation of tissues.

On the other hand, keep in mind that foods rich in complex carbohydrates are much easier to digest and are less calorific than fatty foods, which is why it would be good for you to include a small portion of bread, pasta, or rice, etc. (always whole grain), to maintain the minimum amount of energy your body needs.

At Night, Limit Liquids

Do not drink more than one glass of water (or an infusion without sugar) during dinner to avoid interrupting sleep with the need to get out of bed to urinate. For the same reason, you should avoid diuretic foods at night like celery, onion, or asparagus. While soups or creamed vegetables are appetizing for dinner, they are dishes that contain a lot of liquid and consequently encourage diuresis. At first, this is not necessarily a problem, but, if you are a woman who needs to go to the bathroom very frequently, substitute soup or creams for a plate of grilled, boiled, or salted vegetables.

Ensure Your Dinners Are Rich in Tryptophan

In the evening and night it is good for you to eat foods rich in tryptophan. This compound is an essential amino acid that contributes to increasing the synthesis of serotonin and melatonin, which are neurotransmitters that participate in inducing sleep. Dairies (always fat free), eggs, fish, bananas, meats (always lean), cherries, and nuts (almonds, walnuts, etc.) are some of the foods that are richest in these substances.

Similarly, vitamin B6 and magnesium are necessary micro-nutrients to adequately metabolize tryptophan. This, at the same time, is important for the correct formation of sero-tonin. If your dinner provides a sufficient quantity of both micronutrients, it will contribute to you sleeping better. You will get vitamin B6 from meats (especially chicken or turkey), whole grains, legumes, nuts, wheat germ, and yeast in beer. Magnesium is found in many fruits, whole grains, nuts, and legumes. Avocados and bananas are two fruits especially rich in these nutrients.

Whatever Happens, Eat Dinner

Not eating dinner is a great error. The sensation of hunger acts as a powerful stimulant that can worsen insomnia. It can even provoke you to get up out of bed with an urgent need to snack on something. Additionally, skipping dinner can cause you to suffer nutritional deficiencies, wake up weak and without energy, and, although it seems contradictory, gain weight. Keep in mind that, when you eliminate any meal, the body produces hypoglycemia (it lowers the level of sugar in the blood), which causes you to be hungrier, and therefore, to eat more at the next meal.

The Third Step: Physical Exercise

A routine of moderate exercise, like walking, swimming, running, biking, etc., for at least one hour every day, and preferably in the sunlight, reduces the level of anxiety and increases control over emotional stress. Therefore, in an indirect way it makes you more relaxed and ensures better quality sleep. Additionally, sunlight makes it so that when it comes time to sleep, our body feels the necessity to do so deeply.

Now, if you exercise in the evening, make sure to do so at least five or six hours before going to sleep. If you practice vigorous exercise in the three or four hours before the hour you go to bed, the nervous system can activate itself and then you will lose the sensation of tiredness.

On the other hand, muscular relaxation techniques are also a good option to improve insomnia, just as with hot flashes. For example, Jacobson's progressive method of muscular relaxation has been used and is still used with success to promote sleepiness. Similarly, practicing breathing exercises before going to bed is another relaxation technique that can help you a lot.

To try to have better rest, here is a very simple exercise you could practice: once you are in bed, start to breathe calmly and deeply while you imagine your stomach as a balloon that slowly expands and then deflates. Keep in mind that, during sleep, breathing becomes very deep, regular, and abdominal, so this exercise will help you to sleep better, although it may seem very simple.

Memory Loss and Depression

Mood changes, sadness, and memory problems also form part of the climacteric journey. They do not affect all of us in the same way, but it is quite clear that hormonal imbalance is the trigger of some of the most common psychological symptoms.

Estrogen and other sex hormones are closely related to the brain chemistry involved in our cognition and in our emotional stability. Because of this, hormone swings that are produced throughout this stage sometimes manifest as small lapses in concentration, a low mood, and certain clumsiness in carrying out simple mental tasks, which until now we had been able to do without the slightest problem.

At first, we don't pay attention to this type of change, but when they repeat themselves over time we start to worry, asking ourselves what is happening to us. The truth is that, if we do not have support and the sufficient understanding of these changes, overcoming this rough patch can be hard to manage. Be patient, and above all, do not be scared. As frustrating as it can be, this situation is normal, and when the brain reestablishes its new balance, it will pass.

Memory

Two types of memory exist, one active and another long term. The latter is the one that allows us to remember events that occurred ten weeks, ten months, or ten years ago. On the other hand, short term or active memory is what allows us to manage various facts in our minds at the same time for a few seconds and mix them to be able to elaborate a thought or reasoning. This type of memory has the ability to make us able to work on various ideas, concepts, or data points at the same time.

So, active memory is the one that gives us problems during menopause. Because of this we forget what we were going to say, or the name of the person that we were just introduced to, or the place where we left the keys seconds ago. We have trouble expressing ourselves clearly and quickly though we didn't before entering in this stage.

All of this has much to do with estrogen. This means that blackouts, memory lapses, and difficulties in your cognitive ability are not a sign of Alzheimer's disease or of another type of dementia. This fact is very important to keep in mind because, if you lose sight of it, the doubt that comes from not knowing what is happening to you could generate stress, which would worsen the situation even more.

Little by little, during postmenopause, your cerebral functioning reestablishes itself. That being said, while this occurs, concentrate on doing only one activity at a time. This will make it easier to endure the problem, above all in the work environment.

Estrogen and the Brain

Estrogen stimulates the production of norepinephrine, serotonin, and dopamine. These are neurotransmitters that are involved in memory, learning, mood, and the sleep-wake cycle, among others. This means that these hormones facilitate the communication between neurons, so it could be said that they improve brain functioning.

Because of this, in spite of the fact that it is not completely proven, it would not be surprising if upon an imbalance in estrogen levels there could be fluctuations in the concentrations of said neurotransmitters, and this would lead our cognitive capacity to be affected. In fact, according to a study that was published in the magazine *Menopause*, the first year after menopause is when this problem is exacerbated the most and causes more difficulty with verbal learning, verbal memory, and motor skills. Afterwards, our intellectual capacities normalize and memory loss follows the normal rhythm marked over time.

On the other hand, it is proven that low levels of estrogen are related to the deficit of serotonin, a circumstance which results in changes in mood with a tendency towards negativity. In fact, something very characteristic of the perimenopausal transition, apart from hot flashes, are the ups and downs in mood. In this stage you can feel tremendously dejected and all of a sudden change to a state of excessive anger and irritation. Crying easily is also common, as well as pessimism and feelings of sadness.

The low levels in said neurotransmitter also can produce disruption of sleep, which will vary from one woman to another. Some need to sleep a lot and others cannot at all. When insomnia arises, discouragement and sadness can worsen even more.

It Isn't Just Hormones

The fluctuations in levels of estrogen in some part explain mood changes, mental slowness, and the alteration in sleep patterns.

But, additionally, this hormonal confusion coincides with a very delicate period in our lives. During these years, we tend to live through serious changes in our family lives, with our partner, in our job, and socially, which many times affect us negatively, make us even more vulnerable, and could even decrease our self-esteem. To top it all off, the physical transformation that we experience doesn't help us to cheer ourselves up too much. Because of all this, it is no surprise that we feel sad, confused, and insecure when faced with how to confront our second stage of life.

Uncertain Future

There are also many women who, when they get close to fifty, have the sensation that they have lost something. In the case of some, this feeling of loss can appear alongside the certainty that the possibility to experience motherhood has definitely escaped them. But, in the case of others, it could be that what they feel is the disappearance of motivation, energy, and excitement that until recently were overflowing. Whatever it is, when they think about the direction that they want to take they can get down momentarily. Times arise when they question the future that awaits them and they doubt their capacity to persevere with strength and clarity.

Everything Finds Its Place in the End

Until not long ago, menopause was synonymous with old age and loneliness; in fact, the belief that our personal worth diminishes with menopause is still quite common. However, it is not necessary to think about it much to know that these old ideas are false and do not coincide with reality. Now we live more and better at fifty, we are professionally active, we know how to take care of ourselves, and we have our own projects.

But, although things have changed a lot, the interior crisis that menopause brings us is quite real. It produces nostalgia in us for past times and uncertainty about the future. Now, it is also very true that this stage offers us an opportunity to take a giant step for our evolution. There is no better moment to reconsider our beliefs and customs and reflect upon how we want to live our second life cycle. This step serves us as a trampoline to revive ourselves with more confidence, maturity, and security.

Empty Nest Syndrome

In their forties and fifties, many women watch their children grow up and leave home. This departure produces a sense of loss, disorientation, and sadness, though the woman herself may not readily recognize the root of these feelings. After so many years having dedicated her energy to taking care of the family's wellbeing, when the children leave, so does her reason for being. This experience is what has come to be known as "empty nest syndrome."

With time, the pain passes and leaves room for reflection. This period gives you the opportunity to understand that the moment has arrived to focus your strength on rediscovering and taking care of yourself.

Depression During Menopause

There is no doubt that this period of time demands us to readapt and restructure our priorities. Faced with the uncertainty that the changes generate, it is normal to feel restless and a bit depressed. Now, it is not the same to be in a state of sadness and emotional lability as it is to be in a depressive state.

The combination of hormonal and emotional factors in some especially vulnerable women could cause a depressive state. Those who suffer from noticeable premenstrual syndrome or postpartum depression have a higher tendency to relive the same symptoms (crying easily, fatigue, irritability, etc.) during menopause as a consequence of the influence of estrogen on mood. However, depression in menopause is continuously associated with a feeling of loneliness, uselessness, and low self-esteem, so the factors that influence the emotional sphere are of great importance.

Depression tends to come accompanied by sadness, fatigue, irritability, difficulty concentrating, lack of self-confidence, and insomnia, among other symptoms. But it also affects the way of conceiving reality, which tends to drive a woman towards loss of interest in usual activities and a total indifference towards pleasant moments. This situation impedes following the daily routine and causes suffering, not just in the woman, but in the people around her.

The state of sadness, melancholy, or dejection that arise more commonly during menopause can be combatted with the advice included in this chapter. But if you believe that you have depression, it is recommended that you seek professional help to overcome this challenge in the best way possible. Different therapeutic options currently exist, with or without pharmaceutical treatment, that can help you overcome this situation.

Strengthen Your Brain

Accepting that sadness and memory loss form a normal part of menopause is the first step in calming yourself and going on with higher spirits. But, apart from admitting it, there is a lot you can do to take care of and improve your mental health. Just as with the many physical disturbances that appear in this stage, a healthy lifestyle will help you to protect your cognition.

Do not give up and get going right away. Make the changes to your habits that you need with the objective of stimulating your mind. Keep in mind that diet is fundamental because it will provide the prime material that your brain needs to function. Exercise and breathing techniques are also key. But other activities also exist that are just as important to accelerate and reactivate your brain function. Following are some of the most effective ones.

Fuel Your Brain Well

An unbalanced diet can produce deficiencies of certain nutrients, especially vitamins and minerals, which leads to apathy, irritability, nervousness, fatigue, lack of attention, memory lapses, and even depression. So, to facilitate brain tasks you should begin by watching your diet. To guarantee the contribution of all essential nutrients that your brain needs, your diet needs to be balanced and varied. The nutrients mentioned next are especially important, most of all if you have a predisposition for depression, in which case they should never be missing from your meals.

Basic Energy

The brain represents only 2 percent of our weight; however, it requires around 20 percent of the energy from our diet. An adult brain uses approximately 140 grams of glucose each day; a quantity that can represent up to 50 percent of the total carbohydrates that we ingest. In fact, studies exist that show that a food lacking in this nutrient lowers memory and cognitive capacity, just as others show that consumption of carbohydrates is associated with better mental agility and better concentration and attention as well as a reduction of fatigue.

The explanation of why this happens is simple: glucose is the basic and exclusive fuel that uses the brain to function, and since the brain does not have a way to accumulate it, it needs a constant supply of this nutrient. The best way to ensure a stable level of glucose in the blood is to avoid long periods of fasting and to distribute the diet in five meals, meaning eat less, but more frequently. You should obtain glucose from complex carbohydrates, which are found in whole grains, legumes and potatoes, and in smaller quantities, in fruits and leafy vegetables.

On the other hand, it also benefits you to go without refined sugars. Refined sugars are harmful for general health including mental health. Studies exist that show that a diet rich in refined sugars alters the capacity for learning and memory, as well as causing the brain to work more slowly.

Choose Fats Wisely

Every day more studies show that the consumption of saturated and trans fats is associated with worse cognitive function and long-term memory loss. Similarly, studies also exist that have observed that fats are related to the development of depression. The conclusion is clear: you need to limit the consumption of this type of fat, especially trans fats, which are found in many margarines and in processed foods.

But, while it is good for you to limit the fats mentioned, there are others that you need to include in your diet because they have been proven to have a protective effect on brain function.

✳ Essential Fatty Acids

Omega-3 polyunsaturated fatty acids (linolenic acid, EPA, and DHA) have a positive impact on the protection of good brain functioning. This type of nutrient is a fundamental constituent of the cellular membrane and of myelin, a substance that re-covers nerve endings of the neutrons responsible for brain transmission. Fish, shellfish, and seaweed are the best sources of omega-3 fatty acids (EPA and DHA). Ingesting these foods is associated with better maintenance of brain function.

Another food that contains omega-3 fatty acids, in this case linolenic fatty acid, is the walnut. This nut has the support of studies that have shown the protection that neurons offer when facing oxidative damage produced by free radicals. In the same respect, an investigation carried out by the Clinical Hospital of Barcelona confirmed that consuming between four and seven walnuts daily improves memory of tasks.

✳ Oleic Acid

A high intake of monounsaturated fatty acids, like oleic acid from extra virgin olive oil, helps to conserve cognitive function for more time, thanks to its capacity to slow down mental aging. In other words, regularly ingesting extra virgin olive oil helps to improve memory, learning, attention, thought (capacity for problem solving or abstraction), language, and visual and spatial functioning. Its neutron protecting effect is not only due to oleic acid as previously thought, rather, studies have also attributed it to the antioxidant activity of some of its components, like vitamin E or phenolic compounds.

Vitamins and Minerals

Folic acid and vitamins B6 and B12 improve memory and stimulate correct nervous system functioning, just as antioxidant vitamins C, A, and E. Because of this, a deficiency in these micronutrients is associated with a diminishment in cerebral capacity. Minerals like magnesium, zinc, calcium, iron, and phosphorous, among others, are also essential for assuring good brain functioning.

* Essential Trio

All B vitamins have a specific mission in the conservation of brain functioning and in mental acuteness. Some of them play an important role in the formation of some of the compounds involved in brain communication, like dopamine, epinephrine, and serotonin. The most significant of this group are folic acid and vitamins B6 and B12. In fact, the results of different studies share results that cognitive deterioration is accompanied by their decrease.

Even so, in spite of their confirmed benefits, it is not advisable to take supplements of said vitamins without a medical prescription, since an elevated dose could have a counterproductive effect on your health. Now, it is recommended that you guarantee a good contribution of these micronutrients through your diet. To do so, increase the consumption of vegetables, whole grains, legumes, nuts, lean meats, eggs, and fish, and limit the consumption of alcoholic beverages because alcohol interferes in the absorption of vitamin B1 and can reduce the body's reserves of B12.

* Homocysteine

It is proven that folic acid and vitamins B6 and B12 contribute to the regulation of levels of homocysteine in the blood. This amino acid is produced naturally, but its levels increase over the years. Now we know that the high rates of this compound are related to the deterioration of the blood vessels and the shrinking of the brain. Because of this, the elevated concentration of homocysteine is considered a risk factor for Alzheimer's disease.

Antioxidants

Neuron damage produced by free radicals also affects brain health and causes a weakening in cognitive capacity and memory. One way to reduce oxidative damage is by means of the antioxidants in your diet.

Increasing the consumption of fruits, leafy vegetables, and fresh vegetables is the safest and most effective way to guarantee a good dose of these substances. These vegetables are sources of antioxidant vitamins, like C, E and beta-Carotene, and of minerals with the same effect like zinc or selenium.

But vegetables also contribute many other compounds with the same or even more antioxidant activity. Following are some that have been proven to have the greatest protective effect on the brain.

* Berries for Mental Acuteness

Red berries are especially rich in vitamin C, although they also contain beta-Carotene and vitamins E, B1, B2, B6, and B3. They also contribute minerals like potassium, iron, and calcium and are a good source of fiber. Additionally, these small fruits possess an extraordinary richness in flavonoids, like quercetin and anthocyanin, with antioxidant effects.

According to one of the many studies that has been carried out on these fruits, regularly eating raspberries, blackberries, cranberries, strawberries, etc., helps to maintain mental acuteness and to reduce memory loss. It also seems as though it could manage to delay cognitive impairment that comes with aging and leads to Alzheimer's and other dementias by 2.5 years.

* Grapes for Brain Function and Heart Health

Their composition varies depending on whether they are green or purple. Among the nutrients they contain, the vitamins stand out, especially B6 and folic acid, and in the smallest quantities, they also offer beta-Carotenes and vitamin C. Anthocyanin, flavonoids, and resveratrol are particularly abundant in purple grapes, and are all phytochemical compounds with potent antioxidant action.

Resveratrol is related to better heart health, even has an anti-aging effect, and some studies have shown antitumor properties. But that's not all: various studies exist that suggest that this compound contributes to improving memory and brain function in older people.

✻ Dark Chocolate for a Snack

Dark chocolate also provides a potent antioxidant effect, thanks to its richness in flavonoids, like polyphenols. Their heart-healthy properties are also proven and it seems as though they could favor blood circulation. Although more investigations are necessary to reach conclusions, two studies carried out with this food demonstrated that people who drank two chocolate drinks had increased blood flow to the brain.

On the other hand, one of the polyphenols that chocolate contains is resveratrol, which, as you just saw, appears to contribute to memory enhancement. Now, have just one ounce of dark chocolate (with a high percentage of cocoa and without milk) because, since it is a very calorific food, if you eat more, you will notice it in your weight.

✳ Green Tea's Neuron-Protecting Effect

The popularity of green tea is due to the stimulating effect that it has on the central nervous system. But, apart from this and other beneficial effects, this drink has noticeable antioxidant properties.

With respect to the brain, a growing number of investigations indicate that regular consumption of green tea could delay cerebral aging and reduce the incidence of neurodegenerative disease. For example, one study demonstrates that the combination of an extraction of green tea and theanine improve memory, selective attention, and brain activity in certain zones of the brain.

Theanine is an amino acid with neuron-protecting effects that is present in green tea. Also found in this drink is epigallocatechin-3-gallate (EGCG), a molecule with a potent antioxidant effect with properties very beneficial to the central nervous system.

Most people can drink a few cups of green tea every day without a problem, although it is not recommended in cases of arterial hypertension, cardiac arrhythmias, gastritis, peptic ulcers, epilepsy, hyperthyroidism, anxiety, insomnia, pregnancy, lactation, and in children under twelve years old. What's more, it complicates the absorption of iron from the diet, which is why you should also not drink green tea if you are anemic.

Proteins and Tryptophan

Proteins are necessary for the repair and maintenance of all cells, including brain cells. When they are complete, they contribute all the essential amino acids that we need from our diet because our body cannot produce them by itself. Among these is tryptophan, which functions like a precursor to serotonin, which you already know is a neurotransmitter that favors good mood and better intellectual performance. Said amino acid also facilitates the formation of vitamin B3 or niacin. This being said, protein-filled foods should not be missing from your diet.

Lean red meats, birds, rabbit, fish, eggs, and dairy are animal products that are very rich in proteins that include tryptophan. You can also obtain tryptophan from nuts, whole grains, bananas, and cherries.

Choline

Choline is a substance that intervenes in the transmission of nervous impulse, among other important functions. This compound forms part of the sphingomyelin (found in the myelin that re-covers the neurons) and, from there, the body synthesizes acetylcholine, an essential neurotransmitter for good brain functioning. So, it could be said that choline is a factor that allows brain structures and functions to remain in a good state.

The deficit of this compound can lead to brain dysfunction. However, with a balanced and varied diet it is unlikely that this will happen. In addition to being synthesized by the liver, you can get choline from some fuels like egg yolk, meat, milk, and peanuts.

Exercise Oxygenates the Mind

Regular practice of physical exercise makes you happy, while protecting your cognitive function. Exercise facilitates oxygenation, which means that when you exercise, the quantity of oxygen that gets to the brain increases.

It also seems that exercise allows communication between neurons to be produced more efficiently and fluently. Additionally, physical exercise reduces stress, another of the brain's great enemies. So, it is not strange that those who have incorporated exercise into their lives tend to have better verbal fluency, capacity for reasoning and logical analysis, and better memory, in addition to appearing younger.

But the benefits of physical activity do not end here. Among many other effects, it also activates the secretion of endorphins, which are substances secreted by the brain that act as analgesic and euphoric, and perform a fundamental role in the balance between vitality and depression. An elevated concentration of these substances is related to the sensation of wellbeing, thus physical activity helps you feel better and improves your mood.

Relaxation

Another great enemy of memory and mood is stress. Relaxation is the best method we have to free ourselves of nervous tension. Dedicating a period of time each day to calming yourself will help you to center yourself and to connect with your interior, which leads to better balance, physical as well as mental. Because of this, the practice of relaxation increases vitality and contributes to combatting depression.

In the chapter dedicated to cardiovascular health, you will find a section that includes some tips to combat stress.

Mental Gym to Train the Brain

It is shown that this organ needs to exercise daily in order to offer maximum performance. Because of this, dedicating ten or fifteen minutes to a program of active mental training is priceless, since in addition to having fun, it will help you to have a more agile mind.

There are many techniques designed to exercise memory, concentration, logical reasoning, language, and so on, but you don't have to complicate things too much since training your brain is much simpler than it seems. For example, pastimes like crosswords, Sudoku, and word searches are easy to do, do not take a lot of time, and are effective in keeping your neural circuits in shape. Other games adequate for improving memory and concentration when you are entertaining company are board games like chess, checkers, puzzles, etc. You can also exercise your capacity to pay attention by challenging yourself to focus all you can on something concrete and later make the effort to remember it. For example, you can try to remember the clothing that every one of your work colleagues was wearing or the details of a movie or those of the chapter that you just read in a book.

The Light of the Sun

Sadness and depression can be accentuated in autumn as a consequence of the lack of sunlight. This effect is known as "Seasonal Affective Disorder" (SAD) and although it is a seasonal syndrome whose symptoms will disappear as soon as we adapt to the new season, the sensation of fatigue that it produces can worsen the depression produced by a decrease in estrogen.

The light of the sun influences brain chemistry and modifies the production of the cerebral neurotransmitters serotonin, dopamine, and noradrenaline. Therefore, it is not coincidence that this syndrome aligns with autumn, but rather it is due to the fact that during this cycle, hours of light gradually diminish.

This disorder can be relieved with more exposure to sunlight. Given that the symptoms appear due to lack of brightness and they tend to improve when brightness increases, it goes without mentioning that it is good for you to try to spend more time in contact with sunlight. A simple walk in the fresh air during the sunniest hours of the day will relieve the situation. Another option could be the use of full spectrum lightbulbs at home. These are different than common lightbulbs because they generate a very similar type of luminosity to that of natural light.

Take a Nap

A small nap of fifteen or twenty minutes improves your mood and protects your neural connections. In this time, brain functions rest and recuperate strength from the previous hours. Now, if the nap lasts much longer, it has the contrary effect, as the wake-sleep cycle modifies itself and can lead to or exacerbate insomnia.

Sleep Well

Surely more than once you have gone to sleep with a problem on your mind, and the next day you have awoken with the solution. During the day, the brain collects information and while you sleep it processes and saves it. According to what some studies have shown, one of the essential functions of sleep is the consolidation of the information acquired throughout the day. Rest allows the communication between neurons and the quantity of connections that form between them, and this constitutes the necessary base for learning and memory to last.

But, while rest at night improves brain performance, poor sleeping worsens distractions and mental clumsiness, and even has been related with a higher risk of Alzheimer's disease. Because of this, if you suffer from insomnia, which is unfortunately very common during perimenopause, do not hesitate to seek professional help to solve the problem. The tips to sleep well included in the previous chapter will help you to improve this situation.

Avoid Routine and Stay Active

Always doing things the same way, at the same time, and with the same people not only provokes despondency long-term but also limits our brains, which get settled into convenience. Continuous repetitions do not sit well with the brain since the mind needs to maintain active neural webs to continue learning and feel well-maintained.

The brain learns and activates itself with each small effort that you demand of it. Putting it to the test from time to time is also beneficial. Beginning different mental activities, like studying a language, attending a conference, playing a new instrument, etc., are examples of how to take your mind out of stagnancy and awaken its interest in learning new things. Changing routines and itineraries, such as rearranging the order of domestic tasks or changing the ritual of getting dressed in the morning, also serves to put your mind to the test.

Smoking Damages Neurons

Many investigations have shown that there are up to 4,500 substances in cigarette smoke that are very damaging for our health. Some of them are toxins as well-known as benzo(a)pyrenes, tar, and heavy metals like lead, and even compounds with a high oxidizing power like oxygen radicals and nitrogen oxides and sulfur.

Among their many risks, a French study published in the magazine *Archives of Internal Medicine* affirms that smoking can also cause greater memory deterioration and, consequently, faster progression of dementias. In addition to this investigation, many studies presently exist that reveal that tobacco is a clear risk factor for the development of dementias and Alzheimer's disease.

* And It Makes Depression Worse

The widest long-term study completed at this moment, carried out by researchers from the University of Granada and the Institute of Psychiatry at King's College in London has also confirmed that another consequence of smoking is that it increases the risk of depression.

Maintaining your social life not only revitalizes your mind but also helps you to overcome depression and sadness. Talking to friends of your age who also find themselves experiencing menopause is a good escape route, giving you the opportunity to vocalize your fears and doubts with them, as well as the opportunity to understand that you are not alone.

Meeting new friends, laughing with them, traveling, going out to dinner, etc., also keeps your mind in shape and steers you away from depression. Specifically, what is important is finding happiness and optimism in your life, awakening enthusiasm and curiosity to live new experiences and learn from them.

Medicinal Plants Help Your Mind

Homeopathic medicine relies on some medicinal plants that are useful for treating mild depressive states that occur with lack of energy, lack of concentration, fatigue, and insomnia. Perforate St. John's wort (Hypericum perforatum) stands out among these plants, as well as ginkgo biloba, which has been proven to preserve memory.

* Perforate St. John's Wort

This herbal remedy has an anti-depressive and relaxing effect, which contribute to reducing stress and improving sleep. Its function manifests at least two weeks after initiating the treatment.

Before using it, you should consult a specialist, especially if you are taking other medicines. This medicinal plant is effective, but it can have side-effects. It is a photosensitizer and can interact negatively with some pharmaceuticals. Its use is not advised during pregnancy and lactation.

* Plants with Calming Effects

Plants like passionflower, valerian, lime blossom, orange blossom, or hop are helpful in recuperating lost balance, thanks to their calming effects. They manage to diminish nervousness and anxiety and prevent insomnia. Additionally, their calming effect also relaxes the muscles.

* Ginkgo

Thanks to its vasodilating and venotonic properties, this plant acts on the circulatory system by improving blood circulation. It also contains active principles of antioxidant action, which combat the oxidation of fats that circulate in the blood, contributing to improved microcirculation. Because of this, it helps to protect the brain from lack of blood flow, which is very beneficial in cases of Alzheimer's and other dementias. And, although it is still not proven, the use of ginkgo could also improve memory in healthy people.

It is not recommended to use ginkgo leaves in infusions or in other homemade preparations, since they normally do not contain the necessary concentration to be an effective remedy. Therefore, the most recommended way to take ginkgo is in the form of capsules with the doses already measured, pills, fluid extracts, or tinctures. But remember that before taking it, you should consult a health professional. Exercise extreme caution in cases of arterial hypertension and diabetes, because ginkgo has been associated with brain hemorrhages.

The Genitourinary System and Sexuality

O ther common inconveniences experienced during menopause are problems related to the genitourinary system. On this subject, one of the first things we realize during perimenopause is that our menstrual cycles are becoming irregular. Later, when menopause actually arrives, it would seem that periods are no longer a problem. But just when we think we are free of such inconveniences, disturbances and disorders related to the deterioration of the pelvic floor and vaginal atrophy begin to appear. Despite the fact that this is not a particularly pleasant stage, if you stay firm in your plan to continue taking care of yourself, you will probably be able to keep the disturbances at a minimal level that will not get worse.

Irregular Menstrual Cycles

Having irregularities in menstruation during our reproductive years is more common than we believe. But these irregularities do not tend to have anything to do with those that take place during the last years before the definitive ceasing of the period. As menopause approaches, it is common that the menstrual cycle becomes dysfunctional, which does not appear even close to similar to the pattern that was normal until now. In this respect, many women see that their cycles are shorter and others that their cycles get longer in an absolutely unpredictable way. The bleeding also varies and can be very light or extremely excessive, and even with big clots. What's more, some women can have periods accompanied by uterine pain (cramps).

The reason for this menstrual chaos is the hormonal imbalance that is taking place in our body. For example, in the moments in which there is estrogen predominance, menstrual hemorrhages are more abundant than usual. In fact, it is not strange that these bleedings cause an iron deficiency, which if the case, should be treated adequately.

What Can Be Done?

Irregular menstrual cycles form part of the normal course of perimenopause, and there is no way to prevent them. However, just because this situation is within normalcy does not mean that you should avoid a visit to your gynecologist for a complete exam to confirm that your discomfort is in fact due to menopause. This is important because it is easy to brush off the existence of possible damage that can also produce abundant periods. For example, one of the most frequent illnesses in this stage for many women are myomas or fibermyomas, whose principal symptoms are, precisely, strong periods.

The period of time during which you may live with this menstrual maladjustment may seem eternal. But do not forget that this situation will pass and that in a few years (or maybe it will only take months) it will be over. If you can manage the discomfort, it will always better for your health to be patient and avoid pharmaceutical treatments that are proposed to avoid it. Now, if you suffer periods that are very severe, consult your gynecologist regarding the therapeutic option best suited to your situation.

The most common treatment being used to regulate this symptom is the administration of contraceptives or progesterone. This option is not exempt from very serious risks, but in some cases, it could be preferable to submitting yourself to other more drastic and aggressive therapeutic treatments.

What are Myomas?

Myomas or uterine fibromas are benign gynecological tumors. Around 30 percent of women over thirty have one, and since their growth depends on estrogen, myomas can grow while women have their period. However, once menopause passes, they reduce so much in size that sometimes they even disappear. Myomas can be different sizes, affect different zones of the uterus, and there can be just one or many.

Many women have small or moderate myomas, but since they hardly cause them any problems, they might not recognize their presence. Others know because it is detected in a routine gynecological exam. However, in some women, myomas produce very heavy, painful, and long-lasting periods. They can also provoke abdominal bloating, gas, constipation, frequent need to urinate, or pain or pressure in the pelvis.

Should They Be Treated?

If myomas are small and do not cause symptoms, they do not require treatment. Anyway, in many cases it is wise to conduct clinical tests and regular ultrasound checks to monitor their growth. But, if myomas produce symptoms that are too bothersome, it is probably necessary to treat them. The treatment of myomas depends on their seriousness, the type of myoma, age, and desire to become pregnant. Medicines that are usually used to treat myomas are contraceptives (to control the menstrual cycle), iron supplements (to treat anemia in cases of abundant loss), and non-steroidal anti-inflammatories (to treat pain). But, when pharmaceutical methods are not sufficient, it could be necessary to intervene surgically.

Until very recently, the surgical treatment for myomas that was practiced was the hysterectomy (extraction of the uterus). This operation was performed routinely, and of course, without evaluating whether or not it was truly necessary. Fortunately it is no longer like this and this surgical practice is now considered only as a last resort for very serious cases that do not respond to other techniques. Always keep in mind that before a hysterectomy, other options exist to treat myomas (or get rid of them) that are much less aggressive and do not involve extracting the woman's uterus.

The Secret to Our Wellbeing: Pelvic Health

There is no doubt that disorders related to the pelvic floor present themselves much more frequently when we enter the second phase of our life. However, great controversy exists with regard to its relation to menopause. This is due to the fact that the changes related with the pelvic musculature probably also have a lot to do with the wear and tear that comes with aging.

Whatever it is a consequence of, the reality is that a woman's lower urinary tract and genital system share a common embryological origin. Because of this, the vagina, the bladder, the urethra, and the pelvic floor musculature possess receptors for estrogen and progesterone, which make these structures more sensitive to the action of these hormones. Therefore, when estrogen levels decrease, it produces changes in all of these systems.

The Pelvic Floor

The pelvic floor is formed by a combination of muscles, ligaments, blood vessels, and nerves that are located in the pelvis. This structure closes the abdominal cavity and ensures the support of the bladder, uterus, vagina, and rectum. Its mission is to keep said organs in place, which is of vital importance for them to be able to carry out their functions correctly. The pelvic floor also provides stability to the spine and pelvis.

The drop in estrogen that occurs at menopause leads to a loss of elasticity, tone, and thickness of the pelvic musculature. Evidently, this debilitates the pelvic floor, although this is not the only reason for its deterioration. The decreases and increases in pressure throughout pregnancy and during labor, exercise, or traumas to the pelvic area can also weaken the pelvic floor.

Therefore, if this structure is already debilitated or weakened, upon menopause these women may suffer urinary problems. The most common are frequent infections and inconsistency in urgency as well as strength in flow.

Recurring Urinary Tract Infections

Urinary tract infections are common in women of all ages, although statistics show that they increase with age: approximately between 10 and 15 percent of women over sixty years old suffer frequent urinary tract infections.

Low levels of vaginal estrogen produce a decrease in the flowering of bacteria (primarily made up of lactobacillus) that inhabits and protects this zone. When this occurs, the vaginal pH acid changes, which causes the protection of this area to diminish. This, along with the weakening of the pelvic floor or the presence of urine leaks, increases the risk of suffering recurring urinary tract infections after menopause, for example, cystitis.

Urinary tract infections are very tedious and when they repeat regularly they can become truly torturous. Apart from logical hygienic measures and ingesting abundant quantities of water, treatment tends to consist of taking antibiotics.

Other treatments advised for solving this problem is the vaginal application of estrogen. Estrogen increases the concentration of vaginal lactobacilli flora, which manage to maintain the pH acid and reduce recurring urinary tract infections, but remember that hormonal treatments are not free of risks.

Additionally, an option that is more effective, simple, and absolutely free of side-effects to prevent these infections exists: cranberries.

Cranberries and Preventing Cystitis

The cranberry exerts antiseptic and antibiotic action that is very effective against the germs that cause urinary tract infections. Additionally, in relation to antibiotics used for the treatment of said infections, the cranberry is free of side-effects and presents the advantage of having the capacity to inhibit various bacteria from adhering to the epithelium of the urinary tract, which would explain their efficiency in preventing repetitive urinary tract infections. Just because of this, this fruit should be present in the daily diet of all women with a tendency towards cystitis. But its virtues do not end here; the cranberry also possesses antioxidant properties, reduces the risk of cardiovascular illness, improves peripheral circulation, strengthens the immune system, and has a chemopreventive effect. Keeping these benefits in mind, it becomes very clear that eating cranberries regularly is especially recommended for all postmenopausal women.

Urinary Incontinence

The involuntary loss of urine, even if only a few drops escape, is what is known as "urinary incontinence." This urinary problem is also more frequent with age: it is estimated that it affects approximately 25 percent of women over sixty years of age.

The relation between incontinence and estrogen diminishment is not totally proven; in fact, contradictory results exist. In any case, experts who support the association between the two defend the fact that the decrease in estrogen causes the urinary tract's support system to weaken, which, linked with the gradual deterioration of the urethra and the bladder, lead to the appearance of this uncomfortable change.

Stress incontinence is the most common. In this case, urine escapes upon physical effort that increases intra-abdominal pressure, for example, upon coughing, laughing, or sneezing. This problem sometimes originates during pregnancy or during the postnatal period, but is much more common that it presents itself upon entering menopause.

Urgency incontinence, which is to say, when you need to run out of a room in search of a bathroom upon simply hearing water run, is also frequent. This is due to greater bladder sensibility upon any stimulus, mechanic or nervous, which creates the necessity to urinate, even if the bladder is not completely full.

Getting up a thousand times in the night to urinate is also known as "overactive bladder syndrome." This change is characterized by the sensation of urgency and nocturia (waking up at night to urinate) and can occur with or without incontinence.

The Importance of Strengthening the Pelvic Floor

Urinary incontinence does not represent a serious health problem, however, it exerts a very negative impact on our wellbeing. When we suffer this change, all spheres of our lives appear to be affected. The sensation of not being able to control something as basic as urine has a destructive effect on our self-esteem and increases the risk of suffering depression. A Western University (Canada) study revealed that women with mild or moderate incontinence have a 40 percent higher risk of suffering from depression.

On the other hand, just the idea of leaving home and not having a bathroom close by makes us feel very anxious, so our social relations reduce. They also make personal relations more intimate. And, of course, we live through the work day with great preoccupation due to the fear that a possible escape generates in us. Additionally, incontinence often obliges us to get up many times throughout the night, which also contributes to the deterioration of our night's rest.

However, despite the suffering that incontinence can induce, many women do not seek out a solution to the problem. Many times they do not consult their doctor because of embarrassment, but other times they don't because they believe there is no effective treatment or because they believe that incontinence is a natural disorder due to age. But they are wrong, because incontinence has to do with a very usual change that can be treated.

Now, to live our second life cycle to the fullest and enjoy a good quality of life, it is fundamental that we are conscious of the importance of our pelvic floor. We should take care of it adequately, tone it, and strengthen it in order for it to be able to continue achieving its mission of protection and to not give up when faced with any force.

In caring for the pelvic floor, the most effective method is prevention. To prevent problems, you should watch your diet, pay attention to posture, and practice special exercises oriented towards toning the muscles of that zone.

Kegel Exercises

The pelvic musculature can be exercised at any age, but the sooner you start, the better. Currently we are aware of different routines of exercises aimed to strengthen the muscles of this zone that are tremendously effective. Among these are the popular Kegel exercises.

Dr. Arnold Kegel came up with the routine of exercises that take his name in 1948. The objective of this technique was to strengthen the pelvic floor by completing exercises of contraction with the muscles of this zone. But, since today we know that the pelvic musculature should work as a part of a team with the abdomen, the pelvis, and the spine to prevent incontinence, Dr. Kegel's original technique has been perfected. Because of this, now, in addition to training the muscles of the pelvic floor, they exercise deep abdominal muscles and the position of the pelvis and the vertebrae column are kept in mind.

All pregnant women, before and after giving birth, should practice this type of exercise to prevent possible injuries. But, above all, this exercise should form part of the routine of all of us who find ourselves in perimenopause. Practicing Kegel exercises every day really improves the state of the pelvic floor and not only helps in maintaining control of the sphincter but will also improve your sex life. If you do not have pre-existing problems, five minutes a day are enough to keep the pelvic musculature well-toned.

You will find a lot of information regarding this type of exercise in books on the Internet, where videos on how to complete them are also included. Keep in mind that in order to be really effective, they should be practiced correctly, so if you note any discomfort or it does not seem comfortable to practice them, do not hesitate to consult a specialist for directions. Another option that we have to strengthen the musculature of the pelvic floor is Ben Wa balls or vaginal cones. Although they may seem strange to you, these contraptions are very easy to use and give good results.

In case you already have a problem with urine leaks, do not be afraid or discouraged because you can still improve your situation. This being said, do not delay consulting a qualified professional and beginning exercises immediately. When the muscles of the pelvic floor are already weak, it is possible to strengthen them again through the practice of specific exercises. And, if after these exercises you are not able to control loss of urine, ask the specialist to advise you about the therapeutic option that best suits your situation to be able to find a solution.

Diet Adjustments to Maintain Pelvic Health

In addition to strengthening the pelvic musculature with specific exercises, a healthy and balanced diet is also basic to care for it. Excessive diets, very restrictive diets, drastic changes in weight during menopause, chaotic schedules, etc., are bad habits that manifest in the firmness of body musculature, which will also weaken the strength of the pelvic floor. In the last chapter you will find more information about the diet patterns that are good for you to follow to improve health in this stage. Following is some advice to avoid constipation, because this condition, along with obesity, has an especially detrimental effect on preventing urinary incontinence.

Regulate Intestinal Traffic

Many people believe they have constipation if they do not go to the bathroom every day, but frequency of excretion varies according to the natural rhythm of each intestine. Because of this, it is difficult to define constipation exactly. In any case, it can be considered that when two or more of the following situations take place, there is constipation:

* Going to the bathroom fewer than three times a week
* Excreting with force and difficulty more than 25 percent of the time
* Feces is hard, dry, or scarce
* Sensation of incomplete evacuation of the intestines

Apart from rarely going to the bathroom, chronic constipation also involves making considerable overexertion necessary in order to be able to excrete. Because of this, this condition makes it very challenging to maintain the firmness of the pelvic floor, in addition to being very annoying and tedious. The solution lies with following a schedule for meals (and also for going to the bathroom), staying well-hydrated, and trying to get your body moving more frequently. Eating yogurt every day also helps.

* More Fibrous Meals

Now, the key factor for preventing constipation is fiber. Your daily diet should contribute the necessary quantity for your body to facilitate and regulate the motility of the intestine. Fiber, soluble or insoluble, cannot be digested by the body because it lacks the necessary enzymes to do so (this is why it does not contribute calories). However, the function of this nutrient is essential to improve digestion and intestinal activity. Additionally, it diminishes the risk of suffering other disturbances and creates a sensation of satiation, which helps in controlling appetite.

It is recommended to intake between 25 and 35 grams daily. But be careful! If you haven't eaten fiber until now (or you ate very little), you should not introduce it all of a sudden to your diet. This would be an error that would provoke lots of gas, abdominal bloating, intestinal discomfort, and even could bring on constipation. The way to include fiber in your diet without it making you feel bad is by increasing foods with high quantities of it (fresh fruits and vegetables, whole grains, legumes, and nuts) gradually.

On the other hand, keep in mind that it is not necessary to turn to supplements or foods that are sold as being specifically rich in fiber in order to intake the quantity of fiber that you need. The healthiest way to reach the recommended dose is by means of consuming foods that contain fiber naturally. For example, a plate of garbanzos contains 15 grams of fiber; a plate of spinach, 5 grams; an apple, 3 grams, etc. If you add these quantities, you will see that it is easy to reach 30 grams.

* Drink Water

It is also very important to hydrate yourself correctly, since a diet rich in fiber cannot serve its function without the sufficient quantity of water. Water is not only fundamental for this compound to have its regulating effect, but it also causes lighter bowel movements and elimination with less exertion. In fact, when you do not drink enough, feces becomes hard and dry, which makes excretion much more difficult.

Drink between eight and ten glasses of mineral water throughout the day. Other healthy drinks, like homemade fruit juices, infusions without sugar, or fat-free broths also serve to reach your necessary intake of liquids. Avoid drinking sodas or store-bought juices and alcoholic drinks because they have the opposite effect, meaning, they dehydrate you as a consequence of their high sugar or alcohol content. Additionally, if you abuse this type of drink, your health and your weight will suffer the negative effects.

Another basic way to not suffer constipation is to avoid a sedentary lifestyle. Try to move yourself more; even just with walking or dancing every day you will notice changes in your intestinal rhythm. Additionally, keep in mind that exercise contributes to abdominal musculature development necessary for correct excretion.

Take Caution with Laxatives

The custom of using laxatives to avoid constipation often backfires and aggravates the situation. The fact is, although this type of medicine alleviates the situation momentarily, it makes the intestine weaker in the long-term. When this occurs, a total dependence on the pharmaceutical is created and it becomes difficult not to take laxatives.

Do not fall into the error of using them without a medical prescription. Always consult your doctor before using laxatives to evaluate your particular case.

* *Avoid What Constipates You*

A diet rich in cured cheeses, cold cuts, pre-cooked foods, pizzas, fried food . . . is a diet that is inevitably conducive to constipation (and. obesity). These foods contain a lot of saturated fats and calories, but a small quantity of fiber and water. Now, this doesn't mean that you should restrict all fats. Many foods rich in unsaturated fats like nuts, avocado, and especially virgin olive oil are very healthy and also contribute to combatting constipation. Nuts and avocado contain a good dose of fiber and virgin olive oil has a lubricating effect that is very beneficial for the intestinal tract. Because of this, having a tablespoon of this fat between meals helps when it's time to go to the bathroom.

On the other hand, the excessive use of proteins in diets (high protein diets) is not advisable either, because they tend to be deficient in fiber, and consequently aggravate constipation. Keep in mind that many protein-filled foods are of animal origin.

Don't Let Excess Weight Rule Your Life

Obesity is the enemy of general health. At any age, it is important to prevent, but, during menopause it is even more important to avoid excessive weight gain. Beginning in menopause, the distribution of our body fat changes, and we also have a greater tendency to gain weight. As a result we can get fatter, especially around the middle. The problem is that the excess of abdominal fat compromises health because it increases the risk of developing numerable illnesses. Additionally, having too much stomach fat is another risk factor to provoke or aggravate urinary incontinence.

The explanation of why it is this way is simple. The increase in abdominal fat involves an increase in intra-abdominal pressure on the bladder; the muscles of the pelvic floor become obligated to support a greater load and therefore it is more probable that the support system weakens and fails.

The guidelines in the chapter dedicated to diet will help you learn ways to control weight. In any case, if you suffer from significant excess weight, it is important that you put yourself in the hands of a specialist who can help you lose weight and who can advise you regarding the diet that you should follow.

Posture Is Also Important

Maintaining correct body posture, along with healthy eating and adequate exercise, is also key to keeping the pelvic floor healthy and strong. Keep in mind that, since the spine and the pelvis are totally related, when you keep them correctly aligned (which is to say, that the spine is straight and the pelvis neutral), the activity of this structure increases considerably.

On the other hand, the habit of adopting bad posture not only leads to having spine problems, but also causes the pelvic musculature to weaken. When this occurs, the pelvic floor begins losing its capacity to support and the risk of loss of urine increases.

This situation also creates the possibility of pelvic organs descending due to lack of support (this is known as "vaginal prolapse").

When you are lying down, the pelvic floor is relaxed and should not be supporting too much weight, because its activity is minimal. But, upon getting up, due to the force of gravity the pelvic muscles are activated to support the weight of the abdomen. So, according to your posture while sitting or standing, the extra strain of these muscles will also vary.

So it is very important that you control how you feel. Always keep your spine straight and sit on your ischium, meaning the bones you feel when sitting. If you spend a lot of time sitting because of work or whatever other reason, try to pause frequently to get up in order to avoid remaining in the same position for too long.

You should also keep your spine straight and well-aligned with respect to the pelvis when you are standing. But, above all, monitor your posture when you lift weight. When you lift weight, always do so with your knees bent and without overextending, and do not make sudden movements or adopt forced positions. To reach tall objects that are not at your height, help yourself to benches or cushions to reach without difficulty. Always search for the way to make everything you need accessible without having to force your body.

Menopause Is Not the End of Sexuality

Apart from the debilitation of the pelvic floor, another important change that is produced as a consequence of the drop in estrogen is the general atrophy of the genital apparatus. This brings on some gynecological discomfort like dryness or vaginal burning, which, if not solved in time, can be responsible for the deterioration of our sex lives.

It is estimated that this type of change affects between 10 and 40 percent of postmenopausal women, although its prevalence is not completely well defined, so this percentage could be even greater. This is due to the fact that, although vaginal atrophy is a normal part of menopause, many women do not seek help to solve it. They probably don't because, just as with incontinence, many believe that these changes are an irreversible part of aging. However, this discomfort can be avoided or at least improved, but ignoring it can indeed result in a permanent change.

Dreaded Vaginal Dryness

During the fertile years, the vagina possesses adequate conditions to face the continuous changes of the menstrual cycle without any problems. Additionally, estrogen takes responsibility for conserving the elasticity of the vaginal epithelium and making sure that this lining produces a transparent fluid whose mission is to keep the area well lubricated. All of this guarantees comfortable and pleasurable sexual relations.

Estrogen is also responsible for ensuring that the bacterial flora that inhabits the vagina enjoys good health. And, as you have seen previously, these bacteria contribute to maintaining the pH acid at a level that has a protective effect against the proliferation of pathogenic microorganisms.

However, the situation changes when menopause begins. The fall in estrogen makes the entrance to the vagina fragile as the walls get thinner and become more rigid, causing them to get irritated much more easily. It also causes a diminishment in blood circulation and lubrication, which makes vaginal mucus finer and dryer. All of this can be attributed to the change that the vaginal flora and pH levels produce, which favor the development of vaginal and urinary tract infections.

This situation is what is known as "vaginal dryness," "vaginal atrophy," or "atrophic vaginitis." Its most common symptoms are burning, irritation, and itching in the genital area, burning while urinating, and, as if this weren't enough, it also causes many of us to feel pain when we have sexual relations with penetration (dyspareunia).

Not for nothing, vaginal atrophy is the principal cause of sexual dysfunction in middle-aged women. It is logical that the expectation of an irritating and painful relation diminishes our desire for sex. Evidently, this also leads to a lack of desire and excitation. But, while the hormonal changes provoke alterations in sexual response, menopause does not imply the end of our sexuality. Now, to enjoy full and healthy sexuality in our second life stage we need to learn to adapt ourselves to the changes and, if necessary, seek professional help to solve the problems that may arise.

Treatment for Vaginal Discomfort

Vaginal dryness is a condition that can be controlled and even avoided. A healthy and balanced diet and practicing the Kegel exercises that we just discussed contribute to improving this problem. But, in this case, other treatments tend to be necessary.

With regard to other treatments, many times the simple use of vaginal creams and gels with lubricating or hydrating effects are sufficient. This type of product contains compounds with hydrating effects that form a liquid film that prevents irritation and burning while lubricating the area. Some even help to regenerate damaged vaginal tissue.

In severe cases in which blood is produced upon penetration in addition to just pain, the use of estrogen administered vaginally tends to be necessary. These products should be used for short periods of time (for example, twice a week). Since side-effects and conflicts can present themselves, a specialist should prescribe them to you if necessary, indicating the adequate dose and time of use for you.

Keep in mind that these changes are produced gradually, so do not expect them to all happen overnight (in premature or surgical menopause, it can occur suddenly). Because of this, consult a specialist as soon as you start to feel the first symptoms.

Your sexuality does not have to decline after menopause. Rather, it is a confirmed fact that post menopausal women who maintain an active sex life present lower rates of vaginal atrophy than those who do not have sex.

Other Causes of Decreased Sexual Appetite

The decrease in libido also can be a consequence of some chronic illnesses, of insomnia, or of the regular use of some medicines (such as antidepressants, antihistamines, antihypertensives, tranquilizers, and others).

Lack of Desire Is Temporary

Despite the vaginal inconveniences that can make a sex life more difficult, many women enjoy their sexuality more than ever while in menopause. In this stage they feel less inhibited, they have made peace with their minds and bodies and are no longer burdened by the worry of becoming pregnant. However, many other women do not even want to hear people speak about sex. Now, not having energy for lovemaking is normal, since another consequence of the drop of estrogen is a diminished libido. However, when our desire to have sex fails us, it is not very honest to only blame our hormones. When we find sex unappetizing after menopause, many times there are other causes in play of more importance than our lack of interest. Past conflicts, negative beliefs regarding what is approaching us, a partner who doesn't comfort us anymore, low self-esteem, lack of resources, etc., are only some examples of many issues capable of deflating libido that have nothing to do with hormones.

Apart from the more or less obvious causes, we should also pay attention to the others under the surface that call out to be resolved. Keep in mind that, during menopause, it is common for many thoughts and emotions never before addressed to emerge and develop. Now is a good moment to listen to them and set them free. Working on them will not only make us feel better, but it will also awaken our libido from its lethargy.

Revive Your Sex Life

The second stage of life is a good time to rediscover our sexuality. In postmenopause it is a little more difficult to reach the adequate level of excitement and it takes longer to reach orgasm. But this opens the door to the imagination to dedicate more time to games and caresses and to enjoy more conscious and calmed sexuality. In any case, if you were very worried, lack of excitement can be treated by a specialist. On the other hand, numerous studies indicate that feminine sexual dysfunction in this stage is often related to the partnership. If you have a good emotional relationship, you can maintain your sexual activity for life. Additionally, you can take advantage of this opportunity to encourage communication and get to know each other on a deeper level. Keep in mind that, in postmenopause, your needs could change with regard to what you look for in a partner. Because of this, it is a great time to talk honestly, review the state of your relationship, and work side by side with the objective of re-encountering balance, if necessary. Greater understanding between you both is the secret to affection and rejuvenating an enduring sexual passion.

Prevention of Pregnancy

It is very important during all stages of menopause that you enjoy healthy, controlled, and safe sex. Because of this you will need to use a contraceptive method during perimenopause and continue with it for twelve months postmenopause.

Oral contraceptives are not advisable because of the risk involved. An appropriate method could be condoms. Their effectiveness in the prevention of pregnancy is not as high as other methods (this depends largely on their correct use), but they offer the advantage that they also protect against sexually transmitted diseases.

Healthy, Beautiful, Mature Skin

Something that hurts us, discourages us, and is hard for us to accept is seeing how our skin begins to change. The psychological effect of the state of our skin is really enormous. This organ is our means of nonverbal communication that permits us to relate with others, and naturally, everyone always likes to show their best face. Because of this, we feel bad when we notice the first wrinkles emerge and our muscles are beginning to deteriorate. The media also tortures us with the idea that women above forty enter a decline in which they only have a breath of youth left. It is not surprising that so many perimenopausal women are obsessed with going back in time to recuperate their youthful vitality. But, despite the fact that the belief that beauty is only found in youth is so common, it is absolutely false. Obsessing about it only brings pain and frustration because it is not possible for anyone to stop time.

Never forget that beauty does not reside in your external appearance, but rather comes from inside; it is the pure reflection of how you live and feel about your life. If you feel proud of yourself, of your inner strength, and of your life experience, it is very probable that your attractiveness will accompany you in all periods of your life. Additionally, entering into maturity does not mean entering into old age. Now we have the sufficient knowledge and tools available to navigate this life period and to reach the second half of life feeling better than ever. With regard to the skin, you will keep it healthy and beautiful in accordance with your age if you pamper it and give it the necessary care.

Get to Know Your Skin Better

To know what care your skin needs, it benefits you to know what it is like, how it works, what factors influence its health, and how it transforms as the years pass. This way it will be easier for you to avoid damaging habits that accelerate its deterioration and aging, while you will know how to provide it with everything in your power to help maintain its health longer.

To start, you should know that skin is the biggest organ in the body; in fact, it practically covers it entirely. This allows it to serve as a true physical barrier between the body and the external environment, protecting us from the invasion of microorganisms and other noxious substances. It also plays an important role in the synthesis of vitamin D under the influence of sunlight, it participates in the regulation of body temperature, and it allows the elimination of toxins through sweat.

In the same way that it separates us from the external environment, it also keeps us in permanent contact with it. This is possible because, although it is the most superficial part of the body, it is irrigated by blood vessels and connected to numerous nerve endings that allow it to communicate with the brain at all moments. Thanks to the skin we perceive mechanical, thermal, or tactile stimuli coming from outside: we can notice the heat that fire produces in the same way we feel the softness of a caress or the relaxation that a massage produces in us. Because of this, skin also functions as a faithful indicator of our most intimate feelings. Blushing when you feel embarrassed and getting goosebumps before a big jump are emotional responses that manifest through the skin.

How Does Skin Work?

Regarding its structure, the skin is formed by cells that are arranged in an overlapped and stratified way from the inside out. Inside the skin are three very different layers: the epidermis, the dermis, the subcutaneous tissue (or hypodermis).

The epidermis is the most superficial layer, and it is the only one we can see. It is also the finest and is where the continuous process of regeneration takes place. In its internal part (basal layer) new skin cells are constantly formed that are sent toward the outside as they grow. The most mature cells are drained and die. Once on the surface, these dead cells accumulate forming the stratum corneum (the most external part of the skin). From here, with the touch of time, they are liberated in the form of peeling.

Also found in the basal layer of the epidermis are the cells responsible for synthesizing melanin (melanocytes), which is the substance that provides color; the darker your skin, the greater quantity of melanin it has.

After the epidermis is the dermis. This part is much thicker and is mostly formed by conjunctive tissue. This is composed of collagen and elastin proteins, water, and other substances. Collagen and elastin are the proteins that give the skin its firmness, elasticity, and texture. The blood and lymph vessels, nerve endings, sweat glands, and sebaceous glands, which are joined with the hair follicles, are also found in the dermis.

Lastly, the deepest layer of skin is the subcutaneous fat tissue or hypodermis. This zone is composed largely of fat (more than half the body's fat is found here), and it functions as a real protective cushion for the internal organs when facing blows and other traumas. It also acts as an isolating mantle in facing the external temperature.

The Acid Mantle Protector

The stratum corneum (the most superficial zone of the epidermis) is covered by what is known as the "acid mantle" or "hydrolipidic film" of the skin. In reality, this coating is a fine protective emulsion generated by the secretions of sweat glands and dermal sebaceous. It is formed by water, fat, and natural moisturizing factors and its mission consists of isolating and protecting the skin against external aggression, avoiding loss of water, and preventing infection. It has a slightly acidic pH level (between 4.5 and 5.7) which is very important not to alter. To avoid its alteration, do not bathe or shower excessively, avoid scrubbing yourself with sponges, and do not use soaps or bath gels with an alkaline pH level. In its place, always use hygiene products with a pH of 5.5.

Aging Skin

As time passes, the wear and tear that the body shows is something normal and inevitable. But it is in the skin where the proof of the years is obviously reflected. The skin loses its capacity to retain water and the sweat glands secrete less fat, which makes the protective acid coating diminish. Because of this, if we neglect our skin, we will notice that it has a greater tendency to be dry.

Additionally, as the production of collagen and the elasticity of the dermis diminish, the skin loses its elasticity and firmness, which makes way for the first wrinkles to appear and for the skin to start sagging. After twenty-five years of age, it is calculated that the skin starts to lose collagen (up to 1 percent annually), although there is a lot of variation between women, some can arrive at maturity with a relatively low percentage of this protein (up to 20 percent less). The consequence is finer and thinner skin. The darker your skin, the more collagen and elastin it contains. Because of this, women with white skin have a greater tendency to have wrinkles than those with darker skin.

Another aspect of aging skin is that small injuries take longer to heal. This is due to the fact that the skin is losing its regenerative capacity at the same time that the blood vessels of the skin become more fragile and blood circulation slows.

What Happens to Skin During Menopause

Many receptors for estrogen are found in the skin, and this organ responds to the action of these hormones (it is an estrogen-dependent organ). Because of this, the hormonal variations that are produced during the perimenopausal transition will also be evident in the skin in a negative way. Yes, along with the changes that come with age, the drop in estrogen will accelerate skin aging even more.

During menopause, the skin will lose the majority of collagen (as much as 2.1 percent annually), and the secretion of grease from the sweat glands also will drop sharply. These decreases cause the skin to lose its smoothness and to become more wrinkled and dry. For this same reason, the loss of elasticity, tone, and flexibility will be accentuated, above all in areas that have had the most sun exposure. Because of this, throughout this stage we note that the lower part of the face starts to sag, the texture of the neck changes, and wrinkles become deeper, especially in the areas around the eyes and lips. Additionally, the skin reacts awkwardly to external factors, increasing the risk of injury.

This whole process really sounds awful and pretty frightening. However, when faced with this discouraging panorama, there is a lot you can do for your skin. That being said, so that the course of perimenopause doesn't leave an irreversible mark on your skin, you should take care of it every day to avoid the factors that attack it. With these strategies you will not win the game against aging, but you will manage to slow it down, prevent something worse, and maintain your best-looking skin possible.

Skin's Worst Enemies

Age and estrogen are not the only factors that participate in the aging of the skin. A very stressful or sedentary lifestyle, following an unhealthy diet, drinking alcohol in excess, environmental contamination, and dramatic temperature changes also cause the most extensive organ of the body to debilitate, lose natural moisture, and wrinkle. Now, among all factors that can affect it negatively, the most harmful that can be considered the skin's worst enemies are excessive sun exposure and tobacco. Fortunately, it is conceivable to avoid them.

The Effect of Free Radicals

Before delving into the factors that damage the skin, it is important to talk about free radicals. To know what they are, what effect they have, and how they originate will help you to understand the importance of protecting yourself from the effects they produce, by enriching the diet with antioxidant substances. A great part of the phenomena that occur with aging that lead to the development of degenerative diseases are due to the oxidation of molecules as important as DNA, lipids, or proteins. The process of oxidation (oxidative stress) is intrinsic for every living being, and the free radicals are primarily responsible.

Free radicals are molecules that are very reactive and unstable. To stabilize, they modify molecules around them, provoking the appearance of new radicals. This produces a very harmful chain reaction that does not stop until the antioxidants intervene.

Apart from DNA, these reactive molecules can harm other tissues and cause oxidation to plasmatic lipids, which facilitates the formation of atheromas in the arterial walls. In the case of the skin, free radicals attack the collagen and elastin fibers in the dermis, damaging them. The result is that the skin tissue deteriorates, becomes irregular, and wrinkles form.

A good part of free radicals are produced as a result of the body's normal metabolic activity, which is to say, they originate as a result of breathing or digestion, among others. But another part comes from exogenous sources such as pollution, tobacco, solar radiation, medicines, pesticides, etc.

Our body generates some enzymes with antioxidant effects whose mission is to neutralize oxidation caused by free radicals. They always act together to offer better protection for the different organs and systems. Some of the most outstanding antioxidants are superoxide dismutase, catalase, glutathione peroxidase, and coenzyme Q10.

In any moment, the body is effectively fighting against free radicals. The problem arises when it can no longer generate the necessary antioxidants or when it has to continuously face too high a quantity. When this occurs, the body cannot neutralize such a harmed molecule, so the free radicals are able to harm cellular membrane and damage genetic information, which allows the development of numerous diseases.

Luckily, numerous studies have revealed that some foods, above all those with plant origins, provide us with abundant substances with antioxidant action that helps to protect us against the attacks of free radicals.

Sun, but in Moderation

The sun is a double-edged sword. On one hand, it is essential to live, but on the other, it does us harm. Yes, with the adequate intensity and frequency, it has a great beneficial effect on our body; however, in excess and without adequate means of protection, it becomes the principal aggressor against our skin. Spending time in the sun accelerates skin aging and increases the risk of the development of precancerous or cancerous damage.

Two of the types of ultraviolet radiation that the sun emits are UVB and UVA rays. The first are more intense in the summer, between ten in the morning and four in the afternoon, and can cause erythemas (not melanomas). On the other hand,

UVA rays are present with the same intensity throughout the entire year. These penetrate the skin deeply and the free radicals that generate deteriorate the collagen and the elastin, which produce wrinkles and sagging of the skin. They are also responsible for the spots that appear, above all, on the face, hands, and neckline (notice that these changes in pigmentation tend to produce themselves in the zones most exposed to the sun). This distinctly marks aged skin and tends to worry us a lot, not because it is serious, but because it is very aesthetic (also, it is necessary to keep an eye on them). Skin lightening creams do not manage to eliminate them, so the only option is to prevent them by exposing yourself to the sun with caution and protection. Long-term, the UVA rays also can damage and transform cellular DNA, which significantly increases the risk for the development of skin cancer.

To prevent skin deterioration, it is essential to protect yourself from the sun by applying creams with a sun protection factor (SPF) of 15 or higher, depending on the sensitivity of your skin. You should apply solar protection to all exposed parts of the body every day throughout the year, including in the winter. In summer you should maximize precautions, avoiding exposing yourself to sun in the heat of the day (between ten in the morning and four in the afternoon), using sunglasses, hats, or visors.

So, What's Up with Vitamin D?

If it is true that sun exposure without adequate sun protection accelerates skin aging and accentuates spots, it is also important to keep in mind that to achieve a sufficient level of vitamin D we need to have sun exposure without protection.

There are not too many options to solve this dilemma. Because of this, despite what has been said, you should expose yourself directly to the sun for twenty minutes each day. The best times to do so are first thing in the morning or at the end of the day, when solar radiation is not as dangerous.

Stop Smoking

Another great enemy of the skin is tobacco. Nicotine produces vasoconstriction, meaning it makes the blood vessels contract, which makes blood circulation more difficult.

Because of this, if you smoke, this organ receives less oxygen and other nutrients that it needs for its renewal, which diminishes its regenerative capacity. What's more, tobacco is a producer of free radicals, which, along with the other chemical substances it contains (more than 4,000), damage collagen and elastin. It is not surprising that this product brings on wrinkles at an accelerated rate.

In fact, women smokers have skin that is much more damaged, pale, and wrinkled than those who do not smoke. Its damaging effect extends to general health, but in the specific case of the skin, if you want to take care of it, you have no other option than to abandon this habit.

Dermatologic Care in Maturity

Aside from not smoking and protecting ourselves from excessive sun, when we enter perimenopause, adequate care can do a lot to soften the effects of aging and conserve the good state of our skin. Following, we will explore care habits for treating the most external organ of the body.

But, one warning before we start: do not fall into the common error that, if you use many expensive cosmetics you will achieve better looks and even stop the hands of time. At this age we should already have sufficient experience to know that we cannot expect miracles with the use of these products. Additionally, the skin needs to be clean to be able to breathe, so it is not beneficial to overload it. Now, what you should require of the cosmetics that you choose is that they be effective in keeping the skin healthy, flexible, and luminous. An important point to this end is that the cosmetics you use be of good quality, free of toxic substances, and adequate for your age and type of skin.

The Basic Move: Cleanliness and Toning

The first basic dermatologic care technique is cleanliness. Pollution, remaining makeup, personal secretion like sweat or grease, etc., create a deposit of impurities on the surface of the skin that you should eliminate every day. Water is not usually enough to clean it, so much of the time we need to use soaps, milks, or cleaning lotions that do not alter the skin's pH acidity and that are appropriate for our type of skin. Cleaning the skin excessively is not advisable; if you have dry skin, wash it once a day, and if you have greasy skin, twice. Make the water warm, and remember to always take off makeup before going to sleep.

Next, it is recommended to complement cleaning with toning. Toners tend to have a smoothing and binding purpose whose mission is to close pores. This provides a sensation of wellbeing and leaves the skin prepared to hydrate. Depending on the type of skin, use toners with or without alcohol.

Exfoliation

Exfoliation is a method of deep cleaning that serves to eliminate the dead cells that accumulate in the pores. Doing it once or twice a week (once if you have dry and fine skin; twice if you have greasy skin) is especially recommended beginning in perimenopause because during its course, cellular renovation slows down and dead cells stay on the surface of the epidermis for longer. Amongst the ample variety of exfoliating cosmetics that exist, choose a soft one that includes alpha-hydroxy acids (glycolic acid, lactic acid, citric acid, etc.). This type of compound is especially intended to treat the photo-aging of the skin. But, although you can acquire them without a prescription, it is advisable to seek out medical or pharmaceutical advice so they can recommend the product to you and the concentration most adequate for you.

Hydration

Keeping your skin well hydrated is important at all ages. But, from forty years on, it is of vital importance to conserve your wellbeing. Remember that upon entering perimenopause, the skin becomes finer, dryer, and rougher, so it is in much greater need of daily hydration.

Among the many hydrating cosmetics that exist for mature skin, make sure to choose one of good quality that does not contain damaging components, and if possible, that includes active ingredients with antioxidant properties. Those that contain ingredients that favor the natural production of collagen are also a good option. Some of the compounds that have demonstrated effectiveness in this area are: Ester-C vitamin, alpha-lipoic acid, coenzyme Q10, and tocotrienols (high powered vitamin E).

Diet for Skincare

There is no doubt that dermatological care is essential to preserve your best possible appearance. But this is not enough. Routine moderate exercise and a balanced diet are other crucial factors that will help you to conserve your skin's health during and after menopause.

Exercise is a great ally for the conservation of a good physical and mental state. Among its many benefits, regularly practicing exercise allows the skin to acquire a healthier, fresher, and smoother appearance, because it stimulates blood and lymphatic circulation, which improves oxygenation, the use of nutrients, and the elimination of toxins.

If in addition to exercising you keep yourself well-hydrated and internally well-nourished, there will be more possibility for your appearance to rejuvenate itself. The signs of aging on the face and body can improve, even slow down, with the help of a healthy diet.

Stay Well-Hydrated

You have already seen that to combat the dryness of the skin produced by the decrease in estrogen it is essential to hydrate yourself every day. But, keep in mind that true hydration is produced from the inside. In fact, the shortage of liquids is quickly noticeable in the skin because it is dehydrated, dries out, and loses flexibility. Because of this, just as it is good to use cosmetics to moisturize the skin from the outside, you also need to drink a minimum of eight glasses of water daily to maintain hydration from the inside. Remember that you can also drink other healthy drinks that do not contain sugar.

Fresh fruits and vegetables also hydrate, since they contain a good quantity of water. Additionally, these plants are rich in fiber, minerals, vitamins, and other antioxidant substances that, as you will see if you continue reading, are substances of vital importance to strengthen and protect the skin's health.

Avoid Nutritional Deficiencies

When we suffer a nutritional deficiency as a consequence of stress, an illness, or simply because our diet is unbalanced, it is first noticeable in the skin, the hair, and the nails. The skin is living tissue, so its cells are continuously renewing themselves. The contribution of certain nutrients is necessary for the production of new cells. Because of this, this organ is immediately weakened upon a deficiency in said nutrients, and its deterioration is reflected in its appearance. Those that most influence its health are proteins, essential fatty acids, vitamins A, C, E, and B-complex, and some minerals like iron or zinc. Needless to say, to protect it you should follow a balanced and above all varied diet that provides you with the nutrients you need. Following is a summary of these essential nutrients, and all of them are included in the diet programs that are found in the last chapter.

Proteins

Proteins are key for the firmness and elasticity of the skin because they are the principal component of conjunctive tissue, specifically, collagen and elastin. In maturity, they are totally essential to repair or renovate body tissues. A diet poor in this nutrient will be reflected in weakness in the skin, muscles, and other areas, among other problems that it can provoke.

Foods of animal origin like meats (always lean), fish, eggs, and dairy (preferably nonfat) are good sources. It is also found in legumes, grains, and nuts.

Unsaturated Fatty Acids

According to some investigations, unsaturated fats (polyunsaturated and monounsaturated) protect skin cells. For example, virgin olive oil is rich in oleic acid (as are avocados and almonds) and contributes to restoring its natural level of moisture and confers better elasticity and firmness of the skin. Additionally, it contains vitamin E and polyphenols with antioxidant effects. Because of this, it is good for you to include three tablespoons of this oil every day (not more, to control your weight).

With regard to polyunsaturated fats, regularly ingesting omega-3 acids that can be found in fish (above all blue fish), walnuts, or flax seeds, not only improves the skin's appearance, but also, according to a study published in *The American Journal of Clinical Nutrition*, increases the skins immunity to the effect of sunlight.

Vitamin A or Beta-Carotene

Vitamin A as well as beta-carotene (carotenoid that transforms into vitamin A in the body) have noticeable antioxidant properties. Additionally, they participate actively in the process of cell renewal and are indispensable for regenerating skin, hair, and mucous membranes and for keeping them healthy as a result. In fact, when we do not have enough vitamin A, skin gets dry and rough (especially on the elbows and knees), sweat glands get obstructed, hair dries out and loses shine, and nails become brittle.

Make sure to have the adequate dose of this vitamin by including yellow-orange leafy vegetables and fruits (carrots, pumpkin, mango, peach . . .) and green leafy vegetables (spinach, swiss chard, broccoli . . .) in your daily diet, since they are the foods that contain the greatest quantities of beta-carotene. Sources of vitamin A are eggs, meats, and whole dairy like butter.

Vitamin E

As for vitamin E (which is found in virgin olive oil, nuts, wheat germ, or avocado), this vitamin also contributes to neutralizing the damage of the skin cells from the attack of the free radicals (especially those caused by excess solar radiation).

To ensure you get a good dose of this nutrient, it is enough to eat a little handful of nuts with a drizzle of virgin olive oil to dress them.

Vitamin C

Vitamin C is another substance with antioxidant effects whose presence is obligatory in your diet. This micronutrient is indispensable for the production of collagen. It also promotes the scarring of injuries, stimulates defenses, and facilitates the use of iron coming from other foods. When this vitamin is lacking, problems involving skin dryness and lack of elasticity, among others, are produced.

The sources of this nutrient are fresh fruits and vegetables. Aim to have a minimum of 90mg each day. You will reach this if you have a piece of fresh fruit or a fresh-squeezed juice for breakfast, an assorted salad for lunch, and other fruits for dessert or for midmorning and afternoon snacks.

Complex B Vitamins

B vitamins fulfill a basic role in maintaining good health in this life stage. They are often associated with obtaining energy through metabolic pathways, but also are vital in order to maintain muscle tone and avoid the skin losing its texture and tone. In fact, a deficiency in these vitamins provokes different skin alterations. They are also associated with maintaining the immune system, the cognitive system, memory, and bone health.

Other than vitamin B12, which is found exclusively in animal products, the rest are distributed throughout a variety of products. The best sources are meats, green leafy vegetables, nuts, and some fruits. Beer yeast is very rich in all of these vitamins, so you can add a spoonful of this product to your salads or yogurts to make sure you get the adequate quantity.

The lack of these vitamins can be a result of following an unbalanced diet, having too many sweets and processed foods, or in cases of chronic alcoholism.

Iron

This mineral is essential for the formation of hemoglobin, the component of the blood responsible for transporting oxygen to the whole body. Because of this, when it is lacking, in addition to producing anemia, it causes the skin to become very pale, it increases hair loss, and makes blisters appear in the corners of the mouth.

Your diet will contribute the quantity of iron that you need if you include meats (always lean), eggs, fish, shellfish, legumes, leafy green vegetables, and nuts; and remember that vitamin C increases the absorption of this mineral.

Zinc

One clue regarding the importance of this mineral for skin health is knowing that the majority of zinc in the body is found in the skin, hair, and nails. Zinc is essential for the synthesis of proteins, particularly collagen, and this trace element facilitates the toning and elasticity of the skin.

It also decreases scarring of injuries, and its deficit limits the growth and the regeneration of tissues. Because of this it is used in the treatment of some dermatological disorders and in the scarring process. To guarantee an adequate dose of zinc, your diet should include whole grains, nuts, meat (always lean), fish, and shellfish.

Load Your Meals with Antioxidants

Numerous studies have revealed that a diet rich in antioxidant substances has a protective effect against aging. These components neutralize the damage caused by free radicals, thereby protecting the cell structures. Antioxidants protect general skin health, and the skin improves its firmness and appearance.

Among the antioxidant compounds that you can get through your diet are beta-carotene, vitamin C, and vitamin E, which was mentioned in the previous part. Additionally, foods contain many other compounds with this effect that offer many benefits for skin protection. Some examples are lycopene, which is found in fruits like watermelon or tomatoes; catechins, present in green tea or in cocoa; ellagic acid from pomegranates or strawberries; and anthocyanin from red fruits (cranberries, raspberries, blackberries, etc.). But there are many more.

Because of this, to enrich your diet with these substances you should not obsess about accounting for whether or not you have added this or that vitamin, it is sufficient to increase foods of plant origin to obtain a good quantity of all of them. Fruits, vegetables, and fresh leafy vegetables, as well as nuts, whole grains, legumes, and virgin olive oil are rich in antioxidants.

Are Supplements Necessary?

Taking supplements with antioxidants is a growing trend. You will find them everywhere: pharmacies, diet stores, magazines, books, television, radio, billboards, etc. The reason that we are pushed towards them is the fear of aging.

As you have read in the previous section, it is clear that antioxidants are a great help in conserving a good state of health and slowing down the aging process, but the secret to ensuring their effectiveness is to acquire them through a balanced and varied diet.

Some recent studies indicate that taking supplements with antioxidants not only does not help us but that, when taken in excess, they can do us harm. These same studies confirm that a healthy, daily diet that includes foods rich in antioxidant substances does prove effective. One explanation could include the fact that the supplements only contain one type of antioxidant (or a few more), while foods that are composed of an extensive selection of them act by maximizing each other's strengths. What's more, foods rich in antioxidants tend to be of plant origin, so they also contain water, fiber, vitamins, and minerals.

> If you follow the diet advice that is included not only in this chapter, but in the whole book, your diet will be healthy, balanced, and varied, so you will not need to resort to supplementing with any "extra" products.
>
> In other words, your diet will provide you with all the antioxidants that your skin needs to look its best, to cope with this period of change, and above all, to be healthy.

Lighten Your Diet

The excess of energy in your diet serves as a factory for free radicals. The reason is logical: the more calories we consume, the more our cells will have to work in digestion, and, consequently, more free radicals will be produced. On the other hand, a healthy and light diet will reduce the formation of these attackers and therefore will contribute to slowing the aging process. In fact, according to some authors, the best formula for staying young is to eat a little, but to eat well (underfeeding without malnutrition). But, be careful! Do not confuse a low-calorie diet with a nutrient-deficient diet.

Say No to Sweets and Candies

When you have read every chapter, you will see that limiting foods high in simple sugars and refined flours is repeated as a key point. The list is very long, but some of the most common offenders are pastries and packaged baked goods, cookies, candies, soft drinks, canned juices, etc.

This type of product seriously damages your health in every way. Among other problems, their abuse causes excess weight, dental cavities, an increase in the rate of blood triglycerides, the development of type 2 diabetes, and bone decalcification. It also damages collagen, causing the skin to lose its elasticity.

When we eat too many foods of this type, the levels of blood sugar elevate rapidly. Glucose is the cells' principal source of energy, especially for the nervous system, but its drastic increase causes the pancreas to be strained to produce a greater quantity of insulin to try to manage it correctly. When this occurs, it makes way for very serious health problems. With respect to what concerns us, what occurs when glucose increases all of a sudden is that a small part joins with other proteins, like elastin and collagen. This causes the deterioration of said proteins in a way that the collagen becomes more rigid and loses its flexibility, which ends up producing skin sagging. Because of this, if you want to preserve the firmness of your skin for longer, eliminating sugar from your diet is another way to do so.

Boost Cleansing Processes

In addition to being a barrier that separates us from the outer world, the skin is an organ of elimination. It is known as "the third kidney" for a reason. It participates actively in the body's cleansing processes, and through secretions like sweat, expels waste substances that circulate through the blood to the outer part of the skin.

But, when too many toxins accumulate in the blood, it can exceed the excretory capacity of the skin, which is reflected in worsened skin appearance. Poor functioning of the liver or of the kidneys, chronic constipation, or an unhealthy diet are some possible causes of this situation.

To avoid this, we should facilitate the cleansing processes of our body. To do so, the first step is making sure not to overload it with a diet that is too caloric, or high in sugars, saturated fats, or other damaging substances. At the same time it is good to stimulate the production of urine by abundant water ingestion and by increasing fruits and leafy vegetables, because the majority of them have a diuretic effect and are cleansing. It is also good for avoiding constipation. Intestinal rhythm can be regulated by drinking enough water (1.5–2 liters of water a day) and increasing the quantity of fiber.

Stress Ages Our Skin

Stress decreases blood flow in the skin because it produces vasoconstriction of the venous capillaries, which irrigate the skin. It is also related to the premature aging of cells because it generates a large quantity of free radicals and reduces the efficiency of the immune system. You will find some guidelines that will help you to control stress in the chapter dedicated to cardiovascular health.

Even While You Sleep, Care for Your Skin

Lack of sleep is noticeable in the face and makes the skin seem more tired and less healthy. The reason is that the reparatory mechanisms of the body work during times of rest, so that almost 70 percent of cellular regeneration is produced during sleep. Breathing requires a minimal use of energy and the blood concentrates in the most superficial areas of the body.

In this way, the skin, the nails, and the hair receive more blood flow, which contributes to regenerating them. Because of this, when you sleep enough (between seven and eight hours each night), you allow your skin to recuperate from the damage it has suffered during the day, and that makes you wake up with a better-looking face.

If You're Not Happy with Your Skin, Turn to a Dermatologist

Skin changes in menopause do not affect all women to the same degree. What's more, the impact of the hormonal changes depends on the type of skin of each woman and the lifestyle that she currently lives and has lived. In any case, if you provide your skin the cosmetic care mentioned, you avoid the factors that damage it, and follow a healthy and varied diet, you probably will not have difficulties conserving its health and good appearance.

But, if you had some skin problem that bothers you and that you are not able to improve, do not hesitate to consult a specialist who can evaluate your situation and determine whether or not it is a good idea to use other, more specific resources.

Healthy and Strong Bones for Your Whole Life

Osteoporosis is one of the worst threats that weighs on us after menopause. This condition weakens bones and does not give warning before its arrival; but when it becomes a part of our life, it can weaken our wellbeing tremendously. Not for nothing, it is now considered a great, silent epidemia.

Fortunately, we can do a lot to safeguard our bone health, although to do so we should be conscious of the importance of revising and improving our lifestyle. Following an adequate diet and practicing physical exercise regularly are absolutely necessary to prevent our bones from deteriorating. Staying healthy and strong is priceless because healthy bones permit us to be active and live our lives to the fullest.

Osteoporosis

Osteoporosis means "porous bones" and, as its etymology suggests, has to do with a chronic illness that is characterized by the progressive loss of bone mineral density. As a consequence, the bones become weak and fragile. It tends to happen unannounced, without causing much discomfort, until the first visible sign appears upon small blows or traumas: the fracture. Because of this, it is known as a silent illness.

Nowadays, this bone disorder is more common, and although it can be present in both sexes, it especially affects women after menopause. The fall in estrogen that accompanies menopause leads to a massive loss of bone tissue in a short amount of time. After the loss, it stabilizes and follows a normal rhythm.

What Are the Consequences of Osteoporosis?

Osteoporosis tends to take years to make itself evident, and many times it does so with a first fracture. Because of this, prevention and early diagnosis are fundamental to avoiding its negative effects. Osteoporotic fractures increase with age, and many times lead to a decrease in quality of life. Any bone can suffer a fracture, but the most frequent are those in the wrist, the vertebrae, and the hips.

Hip fractures are the most serious. Their prevalence increases from seventy-five years on, and more than 95 percent of those who suffer them require surgical intervention to repair them. Of these people, fewer than a third will recuperate their normal autonomy. A significant portion of the rest will have an elevated grade of permanent incapacity, and up to 20 percent will die.

Vertebrae fractures are common after sixty-five years. They occur as a consequence of the weakening of the vertebrae. When this occurs, the capacity to be able to support body weight diminishes, and the bones begin to compress. Vertebral crush fractures tend to take place in their internal edge, which produces abnormal forward curvature of the spine. This is known as "kyphosis" and usually takes place in the upper part of the spine. Vertebrae fractures cause diminished height, but also provoke chronic pain as a consequence of the incorrect posture this fracture obligates you to maintain. Additionally, they increase the risk of falls and make many activities of the daily routine more difficult.

With regard to wrist fractures, they are most common in women after fifty-five years. They are not very serious but can be very painful and, if not mended correctly, can cause permanent discomfort.

The Importance of Osteoporosis

Nowadays, osteoporosis is recognized as an important factor in morbidity and mortality. Additionally, osteoporotic fractures involve costly bills for medical services. In fact, according to the World Health Organization (WHO), it is the fifth public health problem at a global level, and it continues increasing. According to a study carried out collaboratively by the WHO and the International Osteoporosis Foundation (IOF) in 2008, "it is expected that the number of hip fractures due to osteoporosis triples in the next 50 years, surpassing 1.7 million in 1990 and up to 6.3 million in 2050."

Faced with this disheartening data, there is no other option than practicing the adequate methods for bone care, without letting another day pass. Keep in mind that with what is referred to as bone health, prevention is the best treatment. In this sense, diet, physical exercise, and sunlight are your best allies.

Risk Factors for Osteoporosis

Two risk factors for osteoporosis that cannot be avoided are age and race: the older you are, the greater bone erosion. In the same respect, Caucasian and Asian women have a greater tendency to suffer osteoporosis than black women. Another risk factor that cannot be avoided is sex. Bone demineralization begins in both sexes at around the age of thirty, but men lose 3 percent of their bone density each decade while women lose 8 percent. In part, this is due to the fact that because our bones are smaller, the effect of wear and tear is greater. But what also greatly influences this figure are the hormonal changes produced during pregnancy and lactation and, above all, during menopause. This is due to the fact that since one of estrogen's missions is similar to bone-forming cells (osteoblasts), when estrogen levels decrease, the process is reversed and causes bone destruction (resorption). But, although age, race, genetics, and being a woman are non-modifiable risk factors, knowing this allows us to be conscious of the importance of adopting more appropriate methods to care for ourselves and prevent this situation.

Now, apart from these inherent aspects of our condition, others exist that correspond to our lifestyle which can be modified to act in favor of our bone health. This section has to do with those that have the greatest impact on our bones—but first, a brief explanation of why it is important to reach a high bone density peak in youth.

Bone Density's Peak

The body is formed of 206 bones that form a rigid structure that is flexible at the same time. This structure is in constant evolution, which means that the bones are created and destroyed constantly. So, their health depends on the balance between both processes: bone formation and bone destruction (resorption).

The most important factor for determining bone strength is bone density. This is determined by the quantity of bone accumulated during growth, and by the following bone loss. So, since bone density increases until reaching its maximum peak in youth, at around twenty to twenty-five years old, there is no doubt that, with the greatest peak reached, there is a greater guarantee of conserving your bones in a good state.

During the period of adulthood, between twenty and forty years old, processes of bone formation and resorption balance themselves, which makes the skeleton appear stable. However, from forty years on, the destruction rate is higher than the formation rate, resulting in the bones beginning to deteriorate. So, when facing the progressive loss of bone mineral density, it is fundamental to have good eating and exercise habits established to keep the bones in good shape.

This is especially important for us because during the five years following the final cease of the period, the loss of bone due to resorption is extremely accentuated. But in addition to the devastating effect of the drop in estrogen levels, women should keep in mind that we tend to reach a lower peak in bone density than men. What's more, in Spain, just as in many other countries, life expectancy has increased. Therefore, if you want to remain upright for your whole life, it is of vital importance that you do all you can to strengthen your bone structure.

What Is Osteopenia?

Osteopenia is an illness that is characterized by low bone mineral density, and on many occasions, it is considered the precursor of osteoporosis. Its early diagnosis is fundamental, because if it is treated in time, this illness is controllable in that it is possible to reverse its effect and avoid more serious bone problems.

Opt for a Healthy Lifestyle

Insufficient nutrients and a sedentary lifestyle are factors that alone could explain bone deterioration and fragility. But there are other factors, like being too thin, smoking, or drinking too much alcohol. All of these should be corrected because they form part of an unhealthy lifestyle.

Unbalanced Diet

Any unbalanced diet is a risk for bone health. Drastic diets for weight loss are also very dangerous. Eating well is basic at any age, but, above all, during childhood and adolescence. In this stage of bone growth people should nourish themselves with all necessary elements for formation to reach maximum bone density. It is also key to ensure adequate nutrition during the perimenopausal transition, in which the bones run an elevated risk of demineralization, as well as in old age. In old age, the body's capacity to reap the benefits of calcium is reduced, so it is also not a good idea to neglect watching your diet. Further along, you will find a part dedicated to how the diet should be to minimize the negative impacts that menopause produces.

Break a Sedentary Lifestyle

Physical activity is an important modulator for bone density in all life phases. Complete immobilization can lead to a 40 percent of bone density loss. Because of this, those who live a sedentary lifestyle are more prone to suffering hip fractures than those who are more active. One data point that clearly proves the importance of breaking the pattern of a sedentary lifestyle is the following: women who remain sedentary for more than nine hours a day are 50 percent more likely to suffer a hip fracture than those who spend less than six hours.

Being Very Thin Is Not Healthy

The relationship between body weight and height helps to give yourself an idea of bone mineral density. Because of this, body mass index (BMI) is of great importance. This variable is one of the most frequently used methods for calculating the degree of thinness or overweight, and it is obtained through the application of the following formula:

$$BMI = Weight\ (lb)/Height^2\ (m^2)$$

The explanation is simple. Since bone is a live tissue that responds to the load that is placed on it, those who have a more elevated BMI tend to present greater bone mineral density. On the other hand, a lower BMI is associated with a greater risk of fracture.

✳ High BMI

The greater the BMI, the greater the bone density. But, according to age and sex, there are differences. In young people and in men, a high BMI tends to be related to a greater proportion of muscle, and since muscle tissue stimulates the formation of bone, bone mass will be greater. However, a high BMI in postmenopausal women is associated with a greater amount of fat, which is to say, with obesity. What occurs is that having a moderate percentage of adipose tissue has a protective effect that helps cushion blows.

Now, although elevated BMIs protect bone health, you should keep in mind that excess weight is not convenient for many reasons. One of them is that being overweight, above all if it is accompanied by a sedentary lifestyle, overloads the skeleton and this can cause serious joint problems. What's more, BMIs greater than 30 are associated with the development of cardiovascular illnesses.

✳ Low BMI

While being overweight is not good, neither is thinness, above all after menopause. Small skeletons present a greater risk of osteoporosis.

✳ Eating Disorders: Anorexia and Bulimia

Eating disorders like anorexia and bulimia can accelerate and aggravate osteoporosis very seriously. It is estimated that between 35 and 50 percent of cases of anorexia present this illness. Extreme weight loss characteristic of these disorders affects the ovaries in a negative way, which stop producing hormones. The deficit of estrogen accelerates the loss of bone density in a similar way to that which occurs during postmenopause. Other factors with influence in these cases are malnutrition and possibly excess exercise, which is often associated with this type of disorder.

Take Care with Alcoholic Beverages

Studies exist that demonstrate that an elevated consumption of alcohol diminishes bone density and significantly increases the risk of fractures. Among other harmful consequences, it is known with certainty that a chronic excess of this substance has a negative impact on bone-forming cells and the hormones that regulate calcium metabolism. What's more, drinking too much alcohol leads to a state of malnutrition and a greater risk of falls.

Recently, studies of populations that drink moderate quantities of beer (one a day for women and two a day for men) have shown that drinking beer in moderation is not harmful for bone health. In fact, said studies found that this drink prevents the loss of bone density. It is suspected that its beneficial effect could be related to its mild estrogenic activity. It could also be that the silicon it contains contributes to said effect.

Tobacco Harms Bones

Smoking is also very harmful for the bones. Tobacco significantly increases the risk of osteoporosis because it causes a decrease in bone density, and consequently increases the risk of fracture, especially after menopause.

Additionally, it slows the scarring of injuries and the healing of fractures. The harmful action of this product increases depending on the quantity smoked during the day and the time smoking.

Medications That Affect Bone Health

Practically all medications present side-effects, but some of them significantly increase the risk of fracture, either because they act negatively against the bone or because they cause a greater tendency for falls. Among the pharmaceuticals that most deteriorate bone health are oral and nasal corticosteroids. Their long-term use is very common due to their anti-inflammatory action, but they present the great inconvenience that their use accelerates the loss of bone mineral density.

Just as counterproductive pharmaceuticals exist for bones, some illnesses also affect them. Among these are malabsorption syndromes like cystic fibrosis and celiac disease. These disorders are associated with a greater risk of osteoporosis as a consequence of the malnutrition that they generate.

In addition to these conditions, others exist that also damage the bone for other reasons. Some examples are inflammatory bowel disease, certain endocrine illnesses, asthma, hypothyroidism, or rheumatoid arthritis.

Early Diagnosis

The greater number of the mentioned risk factors we present, the greater risk we have of suffering osteoporosis. Because of this, if you experience several of these, go to your doctor immediately for a bone density exam. Evidently, you should modify the risk factors that you have that can be avoidable as soon as possible, but additionally, depending on the result of the medical exam, the specialist will advise you as to the preventative or therapeutic measures that best suit your case.

If you do not present any risk factors, it is still a good idea to visit your doctor for an evaluation of your situation. Keep in mind that simply finding yourself in perimenopause is already reason enough for you to take special care of your bones.

Bone Densitometry

Some years ago, osteoporosis was diagnosed by a simple X-ray, and as a result of the limitations of this technique, it was very common for the condition to go unnoticed until the first fracture. Today, this has changed. Now it is possible to detect early bone density loss in the lumbar spine and the hip by dual energy X-ray absorptiometry (DEXA). For now, this tool constitutes the most reliable diagnostic test. It is also a fast and painless test.

The measurement of bone mineral density can be taken in different places, but the most commonly used are the vertebral column between the first and the fourth lumbar vertebrae and the hip.

When Is Bone Densitometry Recommended?

The Spanish Society of Rheumatology justifies performing a bone densitometry exam on women with menopause before forty-five years of age and to those who present one or more risk factors for osteoporosis after menopause (also on men over age seventy). However, many postmenopausal women can present the illness, even without having any of the related risk factors for loss of bone density. Because of this, if you have doubts about your bone health despite living a healthy lifestyle, seek out medical advice.

Other simple exams exist apart from densitometry, like computerized axial tomography (CAT) or certain blood or urine tests, although these are only used in concrete cases and do not tend to be used to diagnose the illness.

Diet and Exercise for Your Bones

Until now we have seen the principal risk factors that aggravate the risk of developing osteoporosis and the importance of early diagnosis. But, upon finding ourselves in the most critical physiological period the bones face, it is not enough to modify the risk factors. We also need to adapt our diet to facilitate the conservation of our bone density and design a new exercise routine focused on not only preserving, but also encouraging conservation of bone density.

Nutrition for Your Bones

The bone is a living and active structure that is forming new tissue and eliminating old tissue throughout your whole life. This process of renovation can be seen affected by nutritional deficiencies and excesses. This is why diet is of such importance in bone health, since the diet provides the basic raw material responsible for forming, maintaining, and repairing bones.

Apart from the widely demonstrated importance of calcium and vitamin D in proper bone formation, currently there is great interest in the effects of a wide range of nutrients and foods that also influence for different reasons.

Generally speaking, to protect bone health, you should increase fruits, vegetables, and seaweed in your diet, moderate the consumption of animal products to the recommended daily servings, and reduce sugar and processed foods rich in refined flours.

A Diet Rich in Calcium

Calcium is the principal component of bones and teeth (99 percent of the body's calcium is found in these structures), and although they perform other important life functions, it is clear that they are indispensable for proper bone mineralization.

An adult person is considered to need 800–1,000 mg of calcium a day. However, there are life stages in which a greater input is required. This is what occurs in menopause, during which women need to intake some 1,500 mg/day.

Daily Calcium Needs

Adolescents	1,200 mg/day
Adults	800 mg/day
Pregnant Women	1,200 mg/day
Menopausal Women	1,500 mg/day
Over 70 Years Old	1,500 mg/day

Dairy

First, to ensure the optimal mineral ingestion, the classic recommendation is to have two to four rations of dairy a day. This recommendation is based on the fact that these products are extraordinary sources of calcium of good bioavailability. Among these, milk, yogurt, and cheese are those that contribute the greatest quantity. But it is better that you opt for nonfat since dairy fat does not benefit us. First, because it is rich in saturated fat, and second because it contains a significant quantity of animal hormones and other compounds that come from its industrialized production.

The same goes for cheeses; they are better fresh and nonfat. Keep in mind that the more treated the product, the more saturated fats it contains, which are associated with the development of cardiovascular illnesses among other problems.

Other Sources of Calcium

Many women cannot or do not want to have dairy. Perhaps because it doesn't sit well with them, because they are vegetarian, or simply because they prefer not to for some other reason. The truth is that there is no problem with calcium if you do without these products. There are many other foods that also contain calcium in addition to other factors (that you will see further on) that influence making better or worse use of it.

Because of this, apart from dairy, you can get the calcium you need from other healthy foods. Moreover, you should rely on them, not only to reach the adequate dose of this mineral, but to also balance your diet. Among those that contain the greatest quantity are small blue fish that are eaten with bones, such as anchovies, sardines, or mackerel. These provide good amounts of calcium and vitamin D, which facilitates calcium absorption.

Legumes (lentils, garbanzos, beans, etc.), nuts (almonds, walnuts, hazelnuts, etc.), seeds (sesame, pumpkin, sunflower, etc.), and leafy green vegetables (chard, spinach, thistle, watercress, cabbage, broccoli, etc.) are also very rich in this nutrient. The inconvenience that these foods present is that, despite being very rich in calcium, it is not taken advantage of like that in dairy. But this problem can be compensated simply by following a diet rich in vegetables. In fact, different observational studies relate a greater consumption of fruit and vegetables with greater bone mineral density. In this sense, another food that can benefit you is seaweed. The richest in this mineral are iziki, wakame, arame, and kombu.

Vitamin D

Vitamin D guarantees good bone health because it facilitates the intestinal absorption of calcium and phosphorous and intervenes in its correct establishment in the bone. Its deficiency leads to rickets, osteomalacia, and osteoporosis, all bone diseases characterized by reduced bone strength.

Apart from being fundamental for correct bone mineralization, the key role that vitamin D plays for general health is growing clearer. Numerous studies have shown that its deficit is related with a greater risk for obesity and the development of cardiovascular illnesses, autoimmune disorders, and even certain types of cancer like colon, breast, or prostate.

The daily requirement of vitamin D is between 400 and 600 IU, but it also varies depending on the physiological stage. For example, pregnant women need 500 IU daily and premature children need up to 1,000 IU daily.

Through our diet we only obtain 10 percent of the vitamin D we need. We get the remaining 90 percent thanks to solar radiation, since our body can synthesize it through the skin. Because of this, it is crucial to get some sun daily to avoid a deficit. In our country, sufficient sun exposure is between fifteen and thirty minutes daily, depending on the hour, the season of the year, and the weather.

In summer, twenty minutes during the hours that are not the hottest of the day is enough. In the winter, the deficit of vitamin D tends to increase 40 percent, so it is beneficial to spend more time outdoors taking advantage of the hours of sunlight. With regard to weather, keep in mind that atmospheric contamination and unfavorable meteorological conditions diminish the formation of this nutrient.

The best would be to get sun on your whole body, but since many times this is not possible, at least make sure that you get sun directly on your face, your hands, and your arms. Something you should keep in mind is that to be able to properly synthesize vitamin D through the skin, you should expose yourself to sun without protection. Sun protection products, despite being necessary to protect us from the harmful effect of excessive sun exposure, present the disadvantage that they inhibit the synthesis of this vitamin.

Personal characteristics also influence the synthesis of vitamin D, since we need more exposure time after fifty years old, if overweight, and if we have dark skin.

To reach a good level of vitamin D it is also important that your diet include some food rich in it every day: blue fish (sardine, mackerel, anchovy, etc.), eggs, or mushrooms. Whole dairy also contains vitamin D, but nonfat does not, since this nutrient is eliminated along with the product's fat. You can also resort to fortified foods. But do not forget that diet alone is not sufficient to satisfy the needs of this vitamin. Because of this, if you cannot sunbathe regularly, consult your doctor to evaluate if it would benefit you to take vitamin D supplements.

Vitamin D Deficiency

Despite the fact that Spain is a country with a considerable amount of hours of sun, it turns out that we do not reach the levels we need of vitamin D (it is the most common nutritional deficiency in the country's population). Various studies that analyzed the diet of women between forty-five and sixty-eight years old concluded that almost 64 percent of the Spanish women of this age did not reach the adequate levels of vitamin D. This fact is of great importance because this deficiency, along with the lack of estrogen, accentuates the risk of suffering from osteoporosis even more.

Proteins Are Also Necessary

Proteins play a binding or forming function for fundamental tissues. Because of this, they are basic for bone formation and maintenance. Not ingesting the adequate quantity of proteins can deteriorate your health. In fact, different epidemiological studies show that diets with low protein contents lead to greater bone loss.

The World Health Organization (WHO) estimates that the protein requirements for an adult person are .8–1 grams of protein per kilogram of weight per day. To reach this recommendation you do not need to make calculations to adjust what you eat. You should simply make sure to include moderate portions of protein-filled foods at least in the three principal meals of the day (breakfast, lunch, and dinner). Now, if you regularly practice a sport at high intensity, you will need a greater quantity (increased to 1.4–1.8 grams per kilo of weight per day).

But, just as eating insufficient protein is harmful, consuming too much is bad for you as well. The excess of protein causes bone decalcification because it provokes a significant loss of calcium through the urine. What's more, it increases the level of uric acid in the blood, which can produce renal damage long-term.

Magnesium

Different investigations have proven that magnesium plays an important role in the balance of the bone, facilitating its growth and stabilization. In fact, more than half of this mineral (65 percent) is concentrated in the bones.

This mineral intervenes in the function of parathormone (a hormone that regulates the balance of calcium and phosphorous) and in the activity of vitamin D, therefore it appears to play a significant role in the regulation of the metabolism of calcium ingested through the diet. Because of this, even if the diet contributes a good quantity of calcium, a magnesium deficiency can lead to its poor absorption, which will make it more difficult for the body to correctly take advantage of its benefits.

For your diet to contribute a good dose of this mineral, you should include nuts, whole grains, legumes, fruits, and vegetables, because they are excellent sources of this micronutrient.

Other Minerals

Despite only needing a very small quantity, other minerals like magnesium, zinc, and boron are also essential for the formation and conservation of the bones. You get boron from fresh fruits and vegetables, nuts, and seeds.

Magnesium comes from legumes whole grains, nuts, green tea, and some leafy vegetables. And good sources of zinc are whole grains, nuts, meat (always lean), fish, and shellfish.

Vitamin K

Vitamin K is known for its participation in blood clotting. Nevertheless, it also intervenes in the production of osteocalcin.

After collagen, it is the second most abundant protein in the bone and appears to play a prominent role in bone mineralization. Recently, it has been suggested that osteocalcin could participate in the control of bone resorption. In fact, according to different studies, a relationship exists between the ingestion of vitamin K and bone mineral density loss: the greater quantity of vitamin K, the lesser the bone mineral density loss.

Its principal sources are leafy green vegetables (spinach, chard, broccoli, lettuce, etc.), and to a lesser extent, whole grains. Since vitamin K is liposoluble (soluble in fats), you will make the best use of it if you consume the foods mentioned above with a fat (for example, virgin olive oil).

Its deficiency is unlikely, because in addition to that which you obtain through your diet, the bacterial flora in the intestine also synthesizes vitamin K and the liver tends to have reserves. In any case, a certain risk exists for loss after long-term treatments with antibiotics in cases of suffering chronic intestinal disease or biliary obstruction and after surgical intervention.

Vitamin C

Vitamin C has a perfectly established role in women during menopause. As you have already seen in the chapter dedicated to the skin, this vitamin is an antioxidant and is essential for forming collagen in the skin, which contributes to maintaining the firmness and smoothness of the skin. But additionally, its deficiency is closely related with osteoarticular problems that often affect us in this stage. A low intake of vitamin C can also be associated with a decrease in bone mineral density at a femoral level. Remember that all fruits, vegetables, and fresh plant products contain it.

Vitamin B12

Vitamin B12 is a necessary factor for the synthesis of DNA and its deficiency produces harmful anemia. What's more, it has been observed that people treated with this vitamin to overcome anemia present an increase in markers of bone formation. It has also been proven that they present an improvement in bone mineral density. As a result of these findings, it is suggested that this nutrient stimulates bone formation because it stimulates the activity of the osteoblasts, although for now the way in which this effect occurs is unknown.

You will obtain the necessary quantity of vitamin B12 if your diet includes the recommended servings of foods of animal origin, which is to say, meats (always lean), fish, eggs, and dairy. In the case of suffering from achlorhydria (deficiency of hydrochloric acid in the gastric juices), common in people of advanced ages, the capacity to absorb said vitamin can be reduced.

Increase Fruits and Vegetables in your Diet

As it has been previously mentioned, different studies have shown a relationship between a greater consumption of fresh fruits and vegetables with a greater bone mineral density. Among other reasons, these plants provide you with high quantities of vitamins, minerals, antioxidants, and other beneficial bioactive components of the bones. But what's more, it is believed that their protective effect is related to their capacity to maintain the body's acid-base balance, since they neutralize the acidifying effect that other foods produce and are consequently harmful for the bones.

For example, you already know that high-protein diets facilitate bone decalcification. The reason is that the metabolism of proteins acidifies the pH of blood, and if the diet does not provide enough alkaline foods (fruits, vegetables, algae), the body will have to resort to the bones' alkaline reserve to neutralize the acidity and to maintain optimum blood pH. This situation will gradually lead to the loss of calcium through the urine and consequently, to bone demineralization.

What Doesn't Help Your Bones

Just as nutrients and foods that benefit bone health exist, there are others that harm it. One of the factors that is most damaging to bone health is a diet with excessive protein, which has been previously mentioned. Following are other eating habits that are also harmful.

Be Cautious with Phosphorous

Along with calcium, phosphorous is an essential element for bone mineralization because it also plays a role in the formation, development, and maintenance of the bones. Other minerals are found in balance in the body, such that when one exists in excess or is lacking, the body's capacity to assimilate is noticeably affected.

It is recommended that the relationship between calcium and phosphorous is 1:1, which is to say, we should consume equal quantities of both minerals. When this relationship is increased to values of 1:2 with more phosphorous, damaging effects begin to present that lead to bone destruction. When this occurs, even if the intake of calcium is sufficient, it could lead to situations of bone demineralization due to the disproportion of these two elements.

Phosphorous is found in many fresh foods that do not pose a problem. But it is also found present in numerous food additives, so if your diet contains many processed foods, it is likely that it causes you to have an elevated ingestion of phosphates. This mineral is also found in carbonated beverages and in cola beverages. In fact, the habit of drinking commercial beverages can facilitate the development of osteoporosis, especially when the ingestion of calcium is low.

Caffeine

Caffeine in high doses produces a slight increase in the loss of calcium and magnesium through urine, but somehow, the body appears to balance out this effect. Available studies regarding this effect conclude that a moderate ingestion of this substance does not have negative effects on young women, since they are able to compensate for the urinary losses with greater absorption. However, women over fifty years old are not capable of compensating for these losses.

This harmful effect acquires a special importance in postmenopausal women whose ingestion of calcium is low. For them, having two or more cups of coffee daily is associated with a greater decrease in bone mineral density. However, those who follow a diet rich in calcium, despite drinking two or three cups of coffee, do not present this problem.

Salt

Although few studies regarding the association between the ingestion of salt (sodium chloride) and bone health exist, an elevated consumption of this condiment is considered to be a risk factor for osteoporosis because it produces an increase in the loss of calcium through the urine.

However, keep in mind that the capacity of potassium to diminish the negative effects of sodium is amply demonstrated.

Consequently, to avoid the use of salt damaging your bones, in addition to reducing table salt as well as from cooking, it also will help to increase fruits and vegetables, since they are excellent sources of potassium.

Physical Exercise Every Day

If you do not use your muscles, they waste away. The same occurs with your bones; if you do not use them, they weaken. Many studies exist that focus on clarifying this fact, but the most conclusive are those that were carried out in the first astronauts after their return from space flight, where there is no gravity.

These investigations could prove very clearly that in the human body after being exposed to the absence of gravity (which is to say that there is no contrasting force to movement), not only was the muscular system noticeably affected, which was weakened and reduced, but also the bones deteriorated to a large degree.

Start Working Out Now

It could be that you don't believe the effectiveness of healthy eating habits or of physical exercise when facing osteoporosis. But it is amply demonstrated that this is how it is. It is a proven fact that frequent, moderate physical activity in postmenopausal women can prevent or revert the loss of bone density almost 1 percent per year. So, take this very seriously, and begin now.

Thanks to these studies, and many more, we now have a better understanding of the relationship between bone density and muscle mass. So it can be said that to provide the necessary mechanical stimulus for the bones, both for development and to prevent damage, physical activity is not enough; the action of the force of gravity is also key.

Therefore, keeping the bone system in shape requires lifting some weight every day. And like muscles, bones respond when subjected to effort. In other words, they are strengthened by supporting more weight than they tend to carry.

Exercise with Weights

Isometric exercises (with progressive resistance) or those that involve supporting weight, contribute to conserving and increasing bone density, which is why they are very advisable for any postmenopausal person. It is a good idea to perform this type of activity three times a week on alternating days.

Even though other types of low-impact exercises without weights, like swimming or bicycling, will not have the same loading effect on the bones, they are still good fitness activities that will keep you in shape. Similarly, yoga and tai chi improve posture, balance, and coordination, which will help you to prevent falls.

Putting an exercise routine into practice in our second life cycle is totally necessary to continue strong and healthily. If you are not accustomed to exercising, adapt the mentality that the moment to move has arrived. It is not difficult to walk some forty-five minutes a day and carry out a routine of exercises with weights three times a week. You don't even have to join a gym because you can do it at home.

Now, if you prefer the option of signing up to a sports center, before starting it is absolutely fundamental that you consult a professional who can evaluate your physical state and advise you on the type of exercise, the frequency, and the intensity most adequate for you. And, when choosing a sport, keep in mind that in order to ensure that you keep your bones in good shape, exercises that are too intense and can also lead to falls are advised against. Excessively aggressive sports are just as harmful for bones as a sedentary lifestyle, since they can cause joint problems and fractures.

Pharmaceutical Treatment of Osteoporosis

If you already have been diagnosed with osteoporosis, you should put yourself in the hands of your doctor to be prescribed the treatment you need and to make you the adequate plan to follow. The principal form of treatment is the use of specific medication to avoid or slow continuous bone loss, or more infrequently, increase bone density. In any case, you should follow a balanced diet rich in calcium and vitamin D, practice regular exercise, and adopt a healthy lifestyle.

A Woman's Heart

Cardiovascular diseases have always been considered to primarily affect men. However, this belief is absolutely false. Currently in Spain, the percentage of women who die from this cause is 8 percent higher than that of men. It is the primary cause of death among western women, well ahead of deaths because of other reasons, such as breast cancer.

Of the almost 65,000 annual female deaths that take place due to heart disease in Spain, 99 percent occur in women over fifty. However, despite the increased risk of cardiovascular disease in postmenopausal women, their relation is not currently totally accepted.

Nevertheless, what we know without a doubt is that estrogen has a protective effect when faced with some cardiovascular risk factors: they are related with low levels of LDL cholesterol (the bad kind) and high levels of HDL (the good kind), they preserve the endothelial function of the arteries, and they thin the blood. The drop in estrogen that menopause produces takes away this protection. Because of this, it is not strange that cardiovascular risk factors also increase.

So believe that heart diseases also affect our life. Once you have that clear, it will be much easier for you to make the adequate changes to adopt a heart-healthy lifestyle that includes not smoking, physical activity, following a healthy diet, and avoiding stress. The sooner you incorporate these healthy habits, the better it will be for your health. Keep in mind that with these simple stops you can diminish your cardiovascular risk by more than 80 percent.

Despite the alarming panorama, the majority of us are not conscious of the fact that cardiovascular illness also has to do with us. The firm belief that these ailments are more common in men probably influences us. In fact, until not long ago, many of the largest studies performed on them didn't even have anything to do with us. Fortunately, now women's cardiovascular health is accounted for just as much as men's. This is how we know that our hearts present differently than those of men. However, these differences are still not very well-known, so many warning signs could pass unnoticed by many women. Since identifying the most common symptoms is a key step to preventing these illnesses, it is of vital importance that you recognize them. Only you will be able to care for yourself as you deserve.

Warning Signs of a Heart Attack

Although pain in the chest or in the left arm can be symptoms of a heart attack in a man, in women, they are neither the only signs nor the most representative. When it happens to us, among the most frequent symptoms are lack of air and discomfort in the chest, which can feel like an ache or pain.

This sensation can extend itself and radiate towards nearby zones like the jaw, the neck, both shoulders, or both arms. Other symptoms that are also common are excess fatigue without apparent reason, unusual anxiety or nervousness, pain in the pit of the stomach, and abdominal discomfort. Similarly, cold sweats, nausea, vomiting, and dizziness can also appear. The great problem is that these symptoms are common during menopause or are usually associated with other conditions, so many times we do not identify them as signs of a serious cardiac problem. This causes us not to pay them the attention they require and, consequently, not seek help. The result is that the woman suffering the heart attack receives medical attention too late. Detecting the symptoms on time and asking for immediate assistance can save your life.

The Importance of Knowing the Risk Factors

Much of the time, cardiovascular illness is diagnosed late, which is to say, when a problem indicating that you are suffering presents itself. For example, arteriosclerosis, which is the most common cardiovascular illness, can begin to develop itself in very early ages. In its initial stages, which last for many years, it does not show any signs or symptoms. In fact, the most serious problem it presents is precisely that it does not clinically manifest during its long gestation period.

When it appears, it does so suddenly so there are no longer possibilities of regression or treatment.

What Is Arteriosclerosis?

This illness consists of the progressive thickening and rigidity of the arterial vessels, which causes a decrease in arterial lumen. This situation leads to worse oxygen and nutrient supply to the whole body. It can eventually obstruct blood circulation and be the cause of serious coronary illnesses.

The repercussion of this process is that when the arteries clog, it gradually can lead to organ ischemia of the organ they supply. In the case of the heart, we can have chest pain or a heart attack; with the carotid artery, a stroke; with the arteries of the lower extremities, it will lead to what is known as peripheral artery disease, which causes us to always have leg pain when walking.

Risk Factors

Without a doubt, prevention is fundamental when facing cardiovascular illnesses. This consists of identifying and modifying the principal associated risk factors. Age and genetics are factors that predispose you to suffering these illnesses that you cannot modify.

However, others exist that are also linked to coronary risk that you can correct to change your course. Among these are smoking, stress, obesity, a sedentary lifestyle, high blood pressure, diabetes, and above all, elevated levels of cholesterol in the blood.

Prevention is important for everyone, but it acquires more importance in perimenopause. In this stage, the majority of us present some of these factors, which is why it is important to find a good professional to carry out a medical revision that includes a cardiovascular evaluation. Keep in mind that the more risk factors you have, the more the possibilities of suffering cardiac problems increase.

In the following parts you will find each of these factors with the most relevant diet advice that will help you avoid them, or if you already suffer the problem, revert it. In any case, remember that in the following chapter you have information that will help you to design your own diet according to all the factors you should keep in mind during and after perimenopause.

Cholesterol: Dangerous yet Essential

As you already know, elevated levels of cholesterol in the blood are harmful and are considered one of the principal cardiovascular risk factors. However, this compound is essential for health, in the adequate quantity.

It is present in the blood and in all body tissues, and forms part of the cellular membrane. It also is the precursor of biliary acids, essential for the digestion of fats, certain hormones like estrogen and progesterone, and vitamin D.

Bad Cholesterol

Cholesterol circulates through the blood joined to something called "lipoproteins." Among these the most commonly known are low-density lipoprotein and high-density lipoprotein. Because of this, cholesterol transported by the first is LDL (or bad cholesterol). LDL cholesterol is produced in the liver, which directs all the cells in the body with the intention to supply oxygen. But when its concentration increases more than what is necessary, it begins to accumulate in the arterial walls. When this occurs, this compound is more susceptible to being oxidized by the action of free radicals.

Oxidized LDL cholesterol is the first step for forming atherosclerotic plaques, whose progression causes atherosclerosis, the most common cause of clogged arteries. Once this process is initiated, the atherosclerotic plaques grow until they can obstruct the regular flow of blood to the vital organs like the heart and the brain, depriving them of oxygen and other vital nutrients for their normal function. Because of this, although it is not alone, an elevated concentration of LDL cholesterol is a cardiovascular risk factor.

Good Cholesterol

The cholesterol that we know as the "good" cholesterol is HDL, and evidently, is that which circulates through the blood with lipoproteins of high density. Its mission is to transport the cholesterol that is found in the tissues (including that which is in the arterial walls) back to the liver, so it can be degraded and eliminated through bile.

Due to the fact that HDL cholesterol has the capacity to remove the LDL cholesterol that is found in the arterial walls, its elevated concentration in the blood is considered to have a cardioprotective effect. Because of this, elevated levels of HDL cholesterol diminish cardiovascular risk.

Ensure That Everything Is in Order

Hypercholesterolemia (high cholesterol) does not present physical signs or symptoms, so it is recommended that you do regular checks with a simple blood test to assure yourself that you have everything in order.

In the case of women, it is considered beneficial to have at least one check before the age of forty-five. But when a risk of suffering an impaired lipid profile or relatives with ischemic heart disease or other cardiovascular disease appears, this test is recommended from early ages.

The concentration of cholesterol in the blood can remain within normalcy simply by following good life habits. To prevent it becoming a problem the only requirements are as easy as eating a balanced diet, regularly practicing physical activity, and avoiding tobacco. Now, if despite these preventative measures your cholesterol levels are above normal, you should seek medical attention to have your specific case evaluated as well as whether or not to prescribe you with an appropriate pharmaceutical treatment.

Cholesterol Levels

Normal values of total cholesterol are estimated to be below 200 mg/dl (milligrams of cholesterol per deciliter of blood). Those between 200 and 239 mg/dl are considered high, and those that go above 240 mg/dl are considered to be a cardiovascular risk-factor.

LDL cholesterol should be below 100 mg/dl, and ideal levels of HDL cholesterol should be above 40 mg/dl in men and more than 50 mg/dl in women. With regard to triglycerides, values lower than 150 mg/dl are considered within normalcy.

Diet to Control Cholesterol

Unless you suffer hypercholesterolemia due to genetics, you can maintain LDL cholesterol levels low and HDL levels high with the help of a diet that is balanced, varied, and low in saturated and trans fats. It should also contain optimum levels of omega-3 fatty acids and lots of fresh fruits and vegetables.

As has already been said, to keep cholesterol levels under control, apart from diet, you should also avoid tobacco, the abuse of alcoholic beverages, and a sedentary lifestyle. Keep in mind that practicing regular moderate physical exercise also contributes to improving your lipid profile.

Heart-Healthy Fats

Currently we all associate high levels of cholesterol with fat in the diet. In part, this is true. But just as it is beneficial to avoid harmful fats, there are also beneficial fats that help us normalize the lipid profile.

Among the problematic ones, we must limit saturated fats, which means that you should reduce fatty meats, cold cuts, full dairy, butter, etc. This recommendation also includes vegetable oils of coconut and palm because they are significant sources of this type of fat. These are found present in many processed products, like pre-cooked dishes, baked goods, and processed cakes.

Trans fats are more harmful than saturated fats and should be avoided. They are found in many margarines and in processed foods like sauces, fried foods, and the already mentioned pre-cooked dishes, bakery products, and processed cakes. You will know that a product contains trans fats when its tag indicates that it contains hydrogenated vegetable fat.

With regard to the cholesterol that food contains, it is not as harmful as it was thought to be some time ago. It appears that when foods rich in cholesterol are abused, only a small increase in the levels of total cholesterol and LDL cholesterol is produced, much less than that caused by the previously mentioned fats. Nevertheless, it is recommended that diets contain less than 300mg of cholesterol a day. This compound is only found in foods of animal origin like meats, fish, shellfish, dairy, and eggs. With respect to the last ones, numerous studies show that despite its high content of cholesterol (200mg/unit), its moderate consumption does not increase cardiovascular risk.

Extra Virgin Olive Oil, Every Day

At the same time as it limits the cited fats, it benefits you to prepare your dishes with simple culinary techniques, like steaming, grilling, or roasting in the oven, and always using extra virgin olive oil for cooking as well as for dressing.

This oil plays a prominent preventative and therapeutic role in the treatment of cardiovascular illnesses. Its star component is oleic acid, which is a monounsaturated fat whose cardioprotective effect is due to its capacity to increase the level of HDL cholesterol, principally. The "extra virgin," which is obtained during the first cold press of the olives, also contains a good dose of vitamin E and other antioxidant components (polyphenols) that help to avoid the oxidation of LDL cholesterol. Because of this, it is a good choice to use this fat every day to decrease cardiovascular risk.

The only inconvenience it presents is its high caloric value, so do not overuse it to control your weight (three tablespoons a day is sufficient). Other foods rich in oleic acid and vitamin E are avocados and almonds.

Blue Fish

A heart healthy diet can also not be missing fish, preferably blue fish. Sardines, anchovies, mackerel, etc., are a source of proteins, vitamins, minerals, and polyunsaturated omega-3 fatty acids (EPA and DHA). This type of fat contributes to reducing cholesterol and triglyceride levels in the blood. But they additionally have anti-inflammatory, antithrombotic, and blood thinning activity, and improve blood pressure. Because of this, blue fish is particularly recommended in the prevention of cardiovascular illnesses. It is recommended to have a minimum of four servings of fish each week, of which at least two of these should be blue.

Nuts and Seeds

Nuts are also very rich in healthy fats (they contain saturated, mono, and polyunsaturated fats in different percentages), as well as minerals, fiber, vitamins, and numerous antioxidant substances. For example, almonds or cashews highlights its percentage in monounsaturated fats, while walnuts and flax seeds are a good source of polyunsaturated omega-3 fats (alpha-linolenic acid). Others, like hazelnuts or sunflower seeds, are especially rich in linolenic acid, which is an essential omega-6 fatty acid. For your diet to be rich in heart healthy fats, it is also beneficial to have 25 grams every day, especially of walnuts or flax seeds.

Now, you should moderate vegetable seed oils, for example that of sunflower or of corn, and use them only occasionally. These fats are rich in omega-6 fatty acids, and although they are essential for health, today we have too much of them. It is ideal to maintain a balance between omega-6 and omega-3; however, our current diet has broken the balance due to a detriment of omega-3. This situation is not at all desirable because the excess of omega-6 facilitates inflammatory processes. This is why the necessity to increase the consumption of foods rich in omega-3 and decrease the consumption of those rich in omega-6 is so important.

Include More Plants in Your Diet

Increasing fresh fruits and vegetables also contributes to controlling cholesterol levels. These plants contribute fiber, vitamins, minerals, antioxidant substances, and other phytonutrients, and all these compounds have a beneficial effect for different reasons. Your diet can also not be missing whole grains or legumes for the same reason.

Fiber from plants contributes to decreasing cholesterol levels in the blood. This is because this compound, above all in the soluble type, acts in the intestine to sequester bile acids, cholesterol, and saturated fats, and promotes their elimination in the feces.

As for antioxidant substances, they are related to hypercholesterolemia because, as different studies have demonstrated, they help prevent the oxidation of LDL cholesterol and thus help reduce the progression of atherosclerosis.

Some of the most well-known antioxidants that these plants contain are vitamins C and E, carotenoids like betacarotene or lycopene, or flavonoids like quercetine or antocianines.

Sterols

Among the many phytonutrients that plants contain are phytosterols or vegetable sterols. These compounds have a very similar structure to that of cholesterol, but they act in the intestine, inhibiting its digestion. Because of this, they have a very positive effect on reducing the concentration of cholesterol in the blood.

Practically all foods of plant origin contain them, but unrefined oils like extra virgin olive oil are those that contain the greatest concentration. Legumes also contribute a good dose, as well as nuts, whole grains, fruits, and leafy green vegetables in a lesser quantity.

An Apple a Day

Having an apple a day (for dessert or midmorning or afternoon snack) provides you with water, fiber, vitamins, and many antioxidant substances. It also satisfies you and contributes very few calories. But, what's more, some studies have demonstrated that some of its components, like pectin (fiber soluble) and polyphenols (antioxidant compounds), contribute to significantly decreasing LDL cholesterol and increasing HDL. This is just an example to give you an idea as to the beneficial power that fruits have on the cardiovascular front.

Whenever you can have a whole fruit, the best way to make the most of all its therapeutic and nutritional richness is raw. In the case of the apple, it also will benefit you in compote or roasted in the oven; it will still be a heart healthy fruit, it will just be more digestive.

Hypertension: Another Surprise Enemy

Blood pressure is the force that the blood exerts on the artery walls upon being driven by the heart: the more difficult it is for the blood to circulate, the more elevated the pressure will be, and consequently, the greater the exertion will be on the heart. Because of this, arterial hypertension is another factor that increases the risk of suffering cardiovascular illnesses.

Since hypertension does not present symptoms either, the only way to know if you have high blood pressure is by means of a regular check. This control will allow you to ensure that your levels remain below the parameters considered acceptable. Much of the time, if they were above the recommended levels, an adequate diet and physical exercise routine is enough to normalize them. But, if that weren't enough to control your blood pressure, you should seek out your doctor's evaluation of the situation.

Control Your Blood Pressure Levels

* **Blood pressure is considered normal when:**

Systolic blood pressure (maximum) is:
   between 120 and 129 mm Hg
Diastolic blood pressure (minimum) is:
   between 80 and 84 mm Hg

* **Blood pressure is considered normal-high when:**

Systolic blood pressure (maximum) is:
   between 130 and 139 mm Hg
Diastolic blood pressure (minimum) is:
   between 80 and 89 mm Hg

What Increases Blood Pressure?

The risk of hypertension increases with age, but it does so in a more pronounced way in women than in men. In fact, after age sixty, it is quite common that we have high blood pressure levels.

On the other hand, its frequency is increased as a consequence of obesity, a sedentary lifestyle, excessive intake of salt through the diet, abuse of alcoholic beverages, and stress.

Blood Pressure and Extra Weight

Arterial hypertension and obesity are related in such a way that it is considered that between 30–65 percent of cases of high blood pressure are due to extra weight. There is no doubt, as your weight increases, pressure levels increase (for every 10 extra kilograms, blood pressure increases 2–3 mm Hg). But, what's more, this occurs with greater frequency in women and in men younger than forty years old. Now, losing weight lowers them, although, if you gain the weight back, the levels increase once again.

The Spanish Society of Hypertension affirms that the only treatment that many people with high blood pressure need to control their levels is losing weight. This means that, whether or not you have high blood pressure, it is very important that you try to control your weight. This recommendation acquires greater importance during perimenopause because as a consequence of the drop in estrogen, we have a greater tendency to gain weight, above all in the central zone. And abdominal fat influences blood pressure in an even more negative way.

If you are overweight, the advice you will find in the following chapter can help you lose weight. But, if it is not enough, put yourself in the hands of a nutritionist right away.

Low-Salt Diet

Sodium intervenes in the control of blood pressure in the regulation of blood volume. This element is also necessary for the transmission of the nervous impulse in muscles and nerves.

When we talk about salt, we immediately think about kitchen salt. Not in vain, as this condiment is sodium chloride, so it contains more than 40 percent sodium. Because of this, recommendations that tend to be made about sodium are expressed in quantities of salt. Without going further, according to the World Health Organization (WHO), we should not have more than 5 grams of salt per day (the equivalent of a levelled teaspoon), which is to say, 2 or 3 grams of sodium. And, in case of hypertension, the quantity should be less, around 1.5 grams of sodium. The reason is that an excess of this mineral causes retention of liquids and increases blood pressure.

But, although we know that it is not good for us to have too much salt, many of us have far beyond the recommended quantity (many times, we duplicate it). Because of this, it is important that we remember that its abuse is a cardiovascular risk factor that can increase the possibility of heart disease and heart attacks. Whether you have high blood pressure or whether you want to take care of yourself, you need to reduce your salt consumption.

Limit the Salt That You See As Well As the Salt You Don't See

To reduce the quantity of salt in your diet, first you should limit how much you use in the kitchen to prepare your meals. And, when you sit down to eat, take the salt shaker off the table so you are not tempted to use it.

Familiarize yourself with aromatic herbs and spices to season your dishes. Other dressings, like lemon juice or garlic, and a good extra virgin olive oil also will help you to not miss it. And, most importantly, avoid turning to commercial sauces and other condiments (soy sauce, tabasco, mayonnaise, etc.) because they are products rich in hidden salt.

You should also limit classically salty products like chips, pickled foods, smoked foods, sausages, cheeses, sauces, etc. Similarly, you should keep in mind that many processed foods contain a high quantity. It is best to get used to eating only fresh and seasonal products and to avoid processed foods, although the truth is that sometimes it is difficult to carry this out. Because of this, if you use packaged foods, before buying them, pay attention to the labels to know what quantities they contribute. The labels tend to indicate the salt content in grams (g). But, if you find one that marks the sodium, remember that it is not equivalent to salt. In this case, an easy way to know how many grams of salt it equals is to multiply the amount by 2.5.

More Fruits and Vegetables

In addition to reducing the quantity of salt in your diet, just as with cholesterol (and cardiovascular health in general), you should reduce saturated fats and increase the presence of fruits and vegetables in your diet to control blood pressure. These plants contain many beneficial nutrients, among them minerals such as potassium, calcium, and magnesium, which have a positive effect on preventing hypertension.

DASH Diet

The DASH diet (Dietary Approaches to Stop Hypertension) is known for its capacity to control blood pressure, without it being necessary to avoid salt. This diet plan also proposes to reduce the ingestion of saturated fat, cholesterol, and simple sugars. Additionally, it emphasizes the importance of increasing the consumption of fruits, leafy vegetables, and nonfat dairy, as well as including whole grains, fish, birds, and nuts because they guarantee the contribution of especially heart healthy nutrients.

Diabetes: An Evil of Our Times

Type 2 Diabetes is a well-known cardiovascular risk factor. It is the most common type of diabetes in adults, and although it currently could be said to be a very common disease, the worst is that its prevalence is predicted to increase even more, above all in developed countries.

This chronic illness involves an abnormal increase in levels of glucose in the blood, in other words, hyperglycemia.

If it is not well controlled, this situation can have serious repercussions. Apart from producing type 2 diabetes, it affects the cardiovascular system because it accelerates arteriosclerosis. Those who suffer type 2 diabetes have two to four more times the probability of developing heart disease than those who do not. But chronic hyperglycemia also increases the risk for osteoporosis because it facilitates bone decalcification; skin health deteriorates, and the risk of developing some types of cancer increases. Similarly, as the years pass, it harms other organs, like the retina of the eyes or the kidneys.

The development of the disorders associated with chronic hyperglycemia is obviously connected to the inadequate control of the disease and the course of its evolution. One of the biggest problems is that if symptoms do not present themselves until a serious complication arises, years can pass before diagnosis. Because of this, prevention is fundamental to avoid the development of this illness and the consequences it entails. Here also, a healthy lifestyle that includes a balanced diet and the practice of physical exercise can achieve your maintained distance from this serious health problem.

Even if you feel well, start today to revise your habits and make the necessary changes to keep your glucose levels constant and within normalcy (between 60–110 mg/dl). This is even more important if you are overweight, if your cholesterol and triglyceride levels are high, if you have a family history of diabetes, and above all, if you are over forty-five years old.

Sugar and Health

Although it seems harmless, having too much sugar can become a very bitter habit: not only do you add a good dose of empty calories to your diet, meaning there is no other nutrient of interest, but you do so in a very unhealthy way that can put your health at risk. Weight gain and a greater risk of developing dental cavities are the most well-known consequences, but sugar's harmful effects go much beyond that. Its excessive consumption also increases the risk of developing type 2 diabetes, heart disease, bone decalcification, and it even facilitates the appearance of certain types of cancer.

When you eat foods rich in sugars and refined flours and lacking fiber, your blood glucose level increases dramatically, and consequently, the pancreas produces a large quantity of insulin. This hormone is responsible for distributing sugar to all the cells, so it can be utilized as fuel. It also orders one part of the glucose to be transformed in glycogen, a compound that accumulates in the liver and the muscles as a reserve of short-term energy. And, when the cells are already well supplied, the same insulin gives the order to convert the extra sugar into fat, which will be stored in adipose tissue cells.

Once the insulin manages to get the sugar to abandon the blood flow, the blood glucose level falls below normal. Therefore, you pass through a hyperglycemic state that causes you to feel tired, irritated, and feel the need to eat more (your brain asks for more sugar). So, it is clear that to calm the sensation of hunger caused by the rapid drop in glucose, you eat again. But you do not eat healthy foods, rather what appeals to you most are carbohydrates, especially sugars and refined products. This causes your pancreas to segregate, once again, a large dose of insulin, and this way, you enter in a vicious cycle that will repeat again and again every few hours, unless you find a remedy.

The problem is that both repeated drastic increases in insulin and excess weight (that probably is a result of eating too much sugar) provoke resistance to insulin (which leads to the development of type 2 diabetes). This means that even if your pancreas produces the sufficient hormones, your body cannot adequately use them because they have a slower, lesser effect. Consequently, glucose cannot pass from the blood to the interior of cells and chronic hyperglycemia (elevated level of glucose in the blood) is produced.

Eliminate Sugar from Your Diet

The consumption of sugar should be very moderate. Since 2002, the recommendation of the World Health Organization is that this nutrient not surpass 10 percent of the total energy of the daily diet (for example, a diet of 1,800 kcal should not have more than 45 grams of sugar). However, this same organization currently is working on a new proposal to reduce the consumption even more to improve the health of the population.

Be Careful with Hidden Sugar

It is possible that you believe you do not have reason to worry about this topic because you consider yourself to not have too much sugar. But, in any case, be careful. Keep in mind that to reduce your consumption it is not enough to limit the quantity that you put in your coffee and avoid sweets, since many other products exist that contain a good dose of hidden sugar, without you suspecting it.

Nowadays, our consumption of sugar tends to be way above what is advisable, but not as a consequence of what we add voluntarily to food, rather because of the large dose that many commonly used processed foods contain. Factories add sugar to their products not only to sweeten it, but also in order to improve the texture of countless products. It is also used to strengthen the flavor of baked goods, sweets, and chocolates, as well as a preservative in marmalades and jellies. Another reason manufacturers use sugar is to facilitate the fermentation of foods like bread and to reduce acidity of those that are made with vinegar or tomato. Unlike that which is present naturally, added sugar to processed products does not have any nutritional value and only contributes empty calories. Because of this, it does not serve you much to eliminate table sugar if you do not restrain from consuming these foods.

Foods with Added Sugars

Soft drinks are one of the products that contain the greatest quantity (one can of whatever soft drink can contain up to the equivalent of six cubes of sugar). So, if you want to take care of yourself, you should abandon the habit of drinking them. At most, you can drink one every now and again.

Cookies, baked goods, ice creams, chocolates, some breakfast cereals, sauces (ketchup, fried tomato, etc.), canned foods, and even commercial fruit juices also contain significant quantities of sugar. It is best for your health to get used to eating fresh, unprocessed foods, and ensure that the only juices you drink are those that you make yourself with the fruits of the season (if you keep the pulp, even better).

Of course, before buying any product, it is essential to read the labels well. For example, syrups and molasses are sugars, although they are disguised with the qualifiers of "healthy" and "natural." In the same sense, many ingredients that end in "-ose" (fructose, dextrose, glucose, sucrose, maltose, etc.) are also sugars.

Sugar, No. Fruit, Yes.

If you are one who believes that since fruits are sweet and contain sugars (above all, fructose), they are not good for diabetics or to control weight, you are not alone. But you are very wrong. Whole fresh fruit, in addition to sugars, contains a good quantity of water, fiber, vitamins, minerals, and other

Healthy Alternative to Sugar: Stevia

The leaves of this plant have an extraordinarily sweet flavor (250–300 times more than table sugar) with the advantage of hardly contributing any calories. It lacks toxicity and different scientific investigations show that its consumption has a positive effect on the control of glycemia and of blood pressure. Another advantage of stevia is that it is set at elevated temperatures, so you can use it for cooking and baking without its properties changing.

antioxidant substances. Fiber slows the absorption of glucose and other sugars, so it reaches the bloodstream slowly and gradually. This does not provoke a sharp rise in blood sugar levels, and it is metabolized slowly.

For example, the difference between drinking a commercial juice or eating a couple apples, is more than just the quantity of sugar, it also has to do with the velocity at which your body assimilates the sugar they contain. The drink is absorbed quickly, so it immediately triggers the glucose rates, forcing the pancreas to secrete a lot of insulin. On the other hand, whole fruit will not produce this effect. In fact, a study published in the magazine *British Medical Journal* found that having fresh fruit can reduce the risk of developing type 2 diabetes.

So do not doubt it, and in order to enjoy something sweet, always choose fresh fruit. They nourish you, they give you energy in a very healthy way, and they take care of your health.

That being said, have them whole. Juices that do not contain fiber because it has been eliminated during the squeezing process are not as beneficial because their GI is higher. Now, you can make them in the blender and preserve this valuable nutrient.

Exercise to Control Sugar Levels

In addition to sugar abuse, a sedentary lifestyle is another factor that predisposes you to type 2 diabetes. Exercise, apart from contributing to burning calories, facilitates insulin action. Because of this, lack of physical activity worsens the resistance to this hormone, above all by muscle tissue.

If you begin to perceive problems with your glucose levels, remember that many times the regular practice of physical exercise along with the adequate hypocaloric diet to lose weight are sufficient measures for the body to return to its balance and for blood sugar levels to normalize.

The Glycemic Index of Foods

The Glycemic Index (GI) is a method that is used to measure the effect that foods rich in carbohydrates cause on blood sugar levels through the process of digestion.

If the GI is high, it means that levels of glucose increase rapidly. This could be harmful, especially for diabetic people. On the other hand, a low GI indicates slower absorption.

Being Overweight: Much More Than a Cardiovascular Risk

It is no secret that eating in excess and not moving yourself sufficiently are intimately related with extra pounds. But, if you are over forty years old and note that your waistline is getting bigger, you are probably gaining weight as a consequence of the hormonal changes that are being produced.

During the course of perimenopause we tend to gain between four and a half and nine pounds (two to four kilograms). What's more, if during our fertile years the fat tended to deposit itself in the hips and gluteus, from now on it will accumulate in the central zone. Up to 25 percent of Spanish women of menopausal age are obese, and in the majority of cases, abdominally obese.

Estrogen and Abdominal Fat

Among other functions, estrogen acts in the brain regulating the sensation of appetite. This is why when its concentration decreases during menopause, it is common that our appetite increases. Its decrease also influences the change in the distribution of body fat. This, along with the decrease of energy expenditure that comes with age, causes us to have a greater tendency to accumulate weight in the central area after the age of forty as a result.

Much More Than an Aesthetic Problem

No one likes gaining weight, and much less, having a belly. However, a larger waistline during menopause is far more than a cosmetic problem. Currently, numerous studies have found that abdominal fat, regardless of whether you have a normal weight, excess weight, or obesity, produces significant metabolic changes in the body. Central fat is an active tissue that generates numerous substances that facilitate the development of the resistance to insulin and type 2 diabetes. It is also evident in the increase of blood pressure and the change of lipid profile, thus having a bulging belly is a very important risk factor when facing cardiovascular illnesses. Another problem that presents itself is that the central adipose tissue has the capacity to produce estrogen. This effect can cause the concentration of these hormones to increase in the blood, which could overstimulate the estrogen-dependent tissues and cause a problem. In fact, abdominal obesity is associated with a greater risk of breast cancer and endometrial cancer. But what's more, having a belly exacerbates hot flashes, urinary incontinence from exertion, joint problems, and as it gets worse, breathing problems.

Measure Your Waist

Whether your weight is within the normal range or you are overweight, you should measure your waist to know if this is your problem or not. Many techniques exist to evaluate the excess of weight, but the waist perimeter is a reliable indicator of cardiovascular risk, as well as for good correlation and its easy measurement.

This method is very useful because, even if body mass index (BMI) is commonly used, sometimes its reading can be misleading. For example, if you are an athlete you will have much more muscle mass and this would make your BMI high without being overweight. However, the waist perimeter does reflect whether or not we have an excess of abdominal fat.

To calculate it the Spanish Society for the Study of Obesity (SSSO) has established the following criteria: you should stand on your feet and use the top of the iliac breast as the reference to measure. Use a tape measure and measure yourself with loose clothes or without clothes.

Values to Establish Cardiovascular Risk
According to the National Institute of Health (NIH)

* For Women

Waist circumference over 32½ inches: moderate risk.

Waist circumference over 34½ inches: high risk.

* For Men

Waist circumference over 37½ inches: moderate risk.

Waist circumference over 40 inches: high risk.

Losing Weight Improves Your Health

Initial weight loss is generally associated with a decrease in abdominal fat, which contributes to improving insulin sensibility and blood pressure levels. Likewise, it tends to produce a decrease in triglyceride and LDL cholesterol levels, as well as an increase in HDL.

Seeing this, you will understand that trying to maintain a normal weight or losing excess weight is of vital importance not only in order to feel more attractive, but also to care for your health. If you do not have too many extra pounds, you will be able to lose them with the diet advice in the following chapter and an adequate physical exercise routine. But, if you are significantly overweight, seek the help of a professional as soon as possible. Most importantly, always remember that losing weight is an achievable goal that can be reached with consistency and tenacity.

Stress Is a Bad Partner

A stressor can be almost anything that causes distress, from toxins in the environment to physical trauma. But what causes us the most stress nowadays is our rhythm of life. Work and family pressures, annoyances, hurrying to get everywhere, etc. tense our nerves every day and undermine our health. But, if we add the hormonal imbalance and contradictory emotions that tend to emerge during the perimenopause phase to the mix, there is no doubt that stress is an important problem that we share with many menopausal women, and that if we do not stop it, it can cause us to see our health very deteriorated.

Nerves and the Heart

When stress does not last long it has a positive effect, because it prepares us to face the challenges that could arise. On the other hand, when it lasts longer than necessary and becomes chronic, stress backfires, heightening fatigue, anxiety, and moodiness that we are probably suffering.

But the damaging effects of being permanently anxious go much further because stress exerts a tremendous strain on many systems of the body, especially the heart, the blood vessels, the kidneys, and the immune system.

Chronic stress is behind the most significant health problems such as digestive disorders, muscular contractions, psoriasis, lack of ovulation, insomnia, or depression and can even facilitate cancerous processes. But with what concerns the heart, it acts as a grand detonator of heart disease: it produces high blood pressure, increases LDL cholesterol levels, and decreases those of HDL. It is also associated with abdominal obesity, worsening diabetes, and on many occasions, leads to addictive habits like smoking, abuse of alcohol, and eating disorders.

Get to Work and Control Your Stress

Whether your heart suffers or not, it is very important that you minimize stress to take care of yourself and successfully overcome perimenopause. It could be that so much is demanded of you by your daily requirements that you do not see it as possible to dedicate some time to yourself to be able to relax. But, even so, you should make an effort to find a way to calm your nerves, because your health is at stake.

The first method to break negativity is to diminish the importance of things. This will not occupy too much time, considering that it has to do with changing the way of seeing life. It is also important to learn to see the positive side of everything and everything that occurs. It seems difficult, but it is a matter of training yourself to get in the habit.

Rest and Laugh

Resting and sleeping well are key. Lack of sleep increases cortisol levels, a hormone involved in stress. Another factor that should not be forgotten about is your social life. Dedicate part of your time to distracting yourself with your friends and laughing together in order to have a psychologically healthy and calmer life.

Laughter facilitates the liberation of endorphins, which are responsible for generating the sensation of wellbeing, and provoking positive effects on the body, such as stimulating the heart, lungs, circulation, and muscular relaxation. What's more, it improves the functioning of the defense system and increases personal satisfaction.

Exercise Every Day

Strengthen your body and your mind to be better prepared to face any situation with more calmness. In this sense, regular exercise has shown its effectiveness to minimize stress and the consequences it involves.

Exercising every day helps you to liberate accumulated tension and allows you to relax. What's more, it increases your energy levels, as well as resistance and capacity to respond when facing stress. Additionally, it improves cardiovascular function because it normalizes cardiac frequency, reduces blood pressure, and decreases levels of cholesterol in the blood, among many other benefits.

Relaxation Techniques, Breathing, and Meditation

Although special methods exist, designed to increase the tolerance and resistance of your mind and body in the presence of stress, other simpler relaxation techniques, breathing, or mediation are also very effective.

Every day more health professionals recognize the benefit of this type of practice, which not only relax, but also improve blood pressure, circulation, and the immune system. With just twenty minutes daily that you dedicate to doing yoga, breathing exercises, stretches, meditation, etc., you can have enough to be calmer.

Diet and Stress

From a nutritional point of view, a healthy and balanced diet designed with the advice that this book includes will serve you as support to combat stress. In this sense, having between five and six servings of whole grains throughout the day is especially important to overcome anxiety. This type of food provides complete carbohydrates that guarantee the constant supply of glucose (the basic and unique brain fuel) in a paused form, avoiding drops in mood.

You should also have foods rich in tryptophan (nonfat dairy, lean meats, fish, bananas, nuts, cherries, etc.). Remember that this essential amino acid contributes to increasing the synthesis of serotonin, a neurotransmitter involved in different moods. Similarly, vitamin B6 and magnesium are necessary micronutrients for the good functioning of the nervous system and the correct formation of serotonin. Nuts, whole grains, and legumes are some of the foods richest in these nutrients, along with bananas and avocados. It could also be good for you to have beer yeast or wheat germ when you are going through a stressful situation.

Medicinal Plants for Anxiety

Just as in the case of insomnia, medicinal plant infusions with a sedative effect contribute to calming the nerves and to relaxing the musculature, which can help you to feel calmer. Some of the most common are valerian, passionflower, linden, orange blossom, or hops. If you so desire, hawthorn is also a good choice.

All these plants are effective and present very few side-effects. In any case, consult an expert about which would be the most appropriate for you before using them.

Tobacco Takes Its Toll

Tobacco does not only affect respiratory tract, but rather all organs of the body, from the skin to the bones. It interferes in hormonal processes and speeds up the date of menopause. And of course, it is also a great cardiovascular risk factor.

The multiple toxic components of smoke act in different ways upon the circulatory system: they diminish levels of HDL cholesterol and increase those of LDL and of triglycerides; they favor thrombosis because they increase plaque aggregation and blood viscosity; they limit the supply of oxygen to the cells, they promote abdominal fat and cause progressive hardening of the arteries, causing arteriosclerosis. What's more, in us women, all these problems can multiply as a consequence of the hormonal changes that are produced in perimenopause.

According to conclusions from the Framingham Heart Study of cardiovascular risk factors, for every ten cigarettes a day smoked, the mortality rate for cardiovascular illness increases 31 percent in women, a percentage much more elevated than that of men, which is 18 percent.

What Do You Gain If You Stop Smoking?

The effects of tobacco on cardiovascular health do not take long to appear. The possibility of suffering a cardiovascular disease is proportional to the number of cigarettes and the number of years during which the habit has been maintained. However, it appears that when you stop smoking, cardiovascular damage reverts itself quickly (it does not occur the same way with other illnesses). Upon reaching one year without smoking, the risk of heart attack decreases by half, and after five years, both the probability of a heart attack or a cerebrovascular accident are the same as those of a non-smoker.

During the twelve hours after smoking a cigarette, the levels of carbon monoxide and nicotine descend and the heart and the lungs to begin to repair the damage caused by the smoke. The benefits of stopping smoking are numerous and immediate: for example, after just a little bit of time maintained without smoking, you will begin to notice that you get tired less easily and you breathe better. It also improves the appearance of your skin and slows its deterioration, recuperates taste and smell, and you cough less.

Stop Smoking. Now.

Quitting smoking is not simple, but if thousands of women have done it, you can too. That being said, to do so, it is important that you are convinced of your decision to stop smoking forever.

Just wanting it is not enough. You should organize yourself, seek out support, and design a plan that helps you pass the first weeks of abstinence. It is important that you avoid situations that you associate with tobacco and that you fill the corners in your environment with trays of fresh fruits and vegetables ready to eat, since they will help you to get through the bad moments when you feel the greatest desire to smoke. Exercise every day, mark a start date to begin your plan, and remember that symptoms of anxiety, nervousness, insomnia, etc., are fleeting and will disappear in two or three weeks.

But, if you believe that you are not capable of quitting smoking alone, do not hesitate to seek professional help. Nowadays, many health centers exist that offer programs of assistance and treatments to quit.

Physical Exercise: A Great Health Ally

As you have seen, exercise is key to maintaining and improving all aspects of health, those that are concerned with menopause as well as those that are more general. And of course, it wouldn't be any less important in what is referred to as cardiovascular health. Physical inactivity is another of the great risk factors for heart disease. If you do not exercise regularly, you run a greater risk of suffering atherosclerosis, arterial hypertension, type 2 diabetes, obesity, and respiratory illnesses. Any person who wants to be healthy and feel good should move more.

There are many benefits of practicing a routine of moderate-intensity exercise every day, or at least four times a week: it increases energy levels, stimulates blood circulation, improves the immune system, controls blood pressure, decreases levels of LDL cholesterol in the blood, prevents osteoporosis, facilitates intestinal transit, etc. There is no doubt that, if your diet is healthy and balanced, you abandon harmful habits, and you move more, you will be able to remain strong and agile, and much more protected against the risk of suffering heart disease.

Cardiovascular Exercise

Cardiovascular exercise is nothing more than aerobic physical activity that makes your heart work. In this sense, the American College of Sports Medicine recommends the practice of aerobic exercise progressively four or five times per week. The recommended duration should be between thirty and sixty minutes per session at a minimum intensity of 60 percent maximum cardiac frequency.

The most adequate outside activities are walking, jogging, bicycling, and dancing. Those that you can do in the gym with a program would be treadmill, elliptical, or stationary bike. It is important that the routine of this type of activity begins gradually, which is to say, from a little to a lot, without overworking yourself and without making too much effort that could lead to muscular or joint injuries.

On the other hand, remember that to avoid muscular and bone tissue loss it is essential to include weight training in your program two or three days a week. Keep in mind that the regular practice of adequate physical exercise is an effective way to remain in good shape, physical as well as psychological, during this life stage.

Break a Sedentary Lifestyle

It is never too late to benefit from physical activity. Sedentary women who begin to exercise improve their cardiovascular health, increase their muscular strength and resistance, and improve their flexibility.

Now, if until this point you have never exercised and you are out of shape, you should consult a professional before beginning to determine the type of activity, duration, and intensity most appropriate for you. A prescription of individualized exercises guarantees that you will be able to improve your situation in a safe way, without running risks. Keep in mind that not exercising is as dangerous for health as suddenly jumping into extreme exercise.

Diet for Menopause

Eating well means a balanced, light, and varied form in which what you eat not only covers all your energetic and nutritional necessities, but also constitutes the sustenance of your health and wellbeing. Now, if your lifestyle currently matches the habits and customs provided, it is more likely that you are not feeding yourself as well as you should, and that menopause won't help.

Reflect and get used to the idea that you will probably have to modify some of your habits. One of the objectives to reach is to relax your rhythm, rest more, and take life more calmly. But it is also key to improve your diet and incorporate an exercise routine into your life. If you adjust your diet in accordance with the advice that this chapter proposes to you, you will cross through the perimenopausal transition without excessive disturbance and the reward will appear.

Soon you will find yourself in a better mood, you will sleep deeply, your skin will improve, and your weight will normalize. What's more, you will be much more prepared to face the disorders that could arise as a consequence of age.

A Light and Balanced Diet

A balanced diet that is low in calories is not only the healthiest and safest way to control weight, but it also ensures that you obtain all the nutrients you need in sufficient quantities to avoid suffering disorders caused by an excess or shortage.

> **The diet is considered to be well-balanced if you have macronutrients distributed in the following way:**
>
> * 45–60 percent of total calories come from carbohydrates
> * 13–15 percent of total calories come from proteins
> * 25–35 percent of total calories come from fats

You should not obsess with counting calories to comply with these recommended percentages. Simply by complying with the following recommendations you will surely manage to adjust your diet so it is balanced. What you should keep in mind is that from now on, since you need less energy, you should have smaller servings of the food that you have been eating until now. A trick that can help you to moderate quantities is to eat on small plates.

Carbohydrates

Carbohydrates constitute the principal source of energy in our diet because during the digestion of these compounds, they divide until they are transformed in glucose, the simplest compound that the body can use as a source of energy. If you reduce its consumption, you imbalance your nutrition.

A balanced diet should supply 45–60 percent of its total caloric value. The problem is the confusion that exists between complex carbohydrates and refined sugars and flours. We should have these others very moderately, or better yet, avoid them totally, because as you have seen in the previous chapter, not only do they facilitate weight gain, but they are associated with many other illnesses. However, our consumption of refined sugars and flours nowadays tends to be higher than what is advisable.

One serving of complex carbohydrates should form part of all meals of the day, above all the three principal (breakfast, lunch, and dinner). Now, if your objective is to lighten your diet to not gain weight, the quantity can be very moderate. You find this nutrient principally in grains (bread, pasta, rice, oats, etc.), but preferably you should choose them from whole grains. Legumes or potatoes are also good sources, but these are better grilled and paired with vegetables.

On the other hand, avoid sweets, baked goods, cakes, soft drinks, and commercial juices, etc. because they are very rich in simple sugars and refined flours which, in excess, will lead you to destabilize your hormone levels even more.

Whole Grains

Opting for whole grains will improve your health and will help you to control your weight more effectively. Although their caloric value is similar to that of their refined equivalents, whole grains provide you with more vitamins and minerals, some beneficial phytonutrients, and a good dose of fiber that will give you the sensation of being full for longer. What's more, they have a lower glucose index than refined equivalents. Because of this, whole grain foods provide you with the energy you need gradually, avoiding drastic fluctuations in levels of sugar in the blood.

Fiber

Although it is not considered a nutrient, fiber is a fundamental component of any balanced diet. Among other benefits, it improves digestion and intestinal transit (so it prevents constipation) and contributes to diminishing the risk of many complications that can develop after menopause (heart disease, diabetes, certain types of cancer like breast and colon, etc.). What's more, it provides the sensation of satisfaction, which helps you to better control your appetite.

It is recommended to have between 25 and 35 grams daily. You can obtain this quantity by including fruits, vegetables, whole grains, and a handful of nuts every day. You should also include legumes three or four times a week. For example, if you have three pieces of fruit a day, two servings of vegetables (a salad at lunch and a plate of chard for dinner), whole grain bread instead of white, and a handful of walnuts, it is very easy to reach this objective.

Proteins

Proteins have many important functions, but what's more, they are the principal component of conjunctive cartilage and bone tissue (collagen and elastin), and they provide strength, elasticity, and protection for the body. A balanced diet is considered to supply between 13 and 15 percent of the diet's total energy. Although, in overweight cases, a hypocaloric diet can have more, between 15 and 20 percent of the total energy value (a diet of 1,800 kcal would have 67.5–90 grams of protein a day).

You should include a moderate serving of some protein-filled food at least in the three main meals of the day (breakfast, lunch, and dinner). You can get them from foods of animal and plant origin. Among meats, fish, dairy, and eggs, the best choice is fish because it also contributes omega-3 oils, minerals, vitamins, and not too many calories.

Eggs contribute complete proteins, vitamins, minerals, antioxidants, and fats. In fact, until not long ago, their consumption was related to high levels of cholesterol due to the fact that it is one of the nutrients that they contain in the greatest quantity (a medium-sized egg of 50g contains some 200mg of cholesterol). Because of this, as a means of cardiovascular prevention, it was recommended to limit consumption to three or four a week, and their consumption decreased. However, now, many studies have shown that the cholesterol that eggs contain hardly influences hypercholesterolemia. What it does increase is the excess of trans and saturated fats.

With regard to meat, it principally contributes proteins, vitamins from the B group (including B12), and iron. But it is also a source of saturated fats, cholesterol, and many calories. Consequently, its excessive consumption leads to a greater risk of suffering heart disease, among other disorders. Therefore, you should have them in moderation. What's more, you should always accompany them with a good serving of leafy green vegetables. Among red and white (chicken, rabbit, turkey, etc.) choose the second, because it has less fat and consequently significantly fewer calories. Now, it is recommended that you cook with simple culinary techniques like the grill or the oven. Frying or battering greatly increases their energetic value.

Those of plant origin that are found in nuts, whole grains, and legumes have the inconvenience that they do not contain all essential amino acids, so to complete the protein content you should always combine them among themselves (for example, whole grains with legumes). Now, they present the advantage that they do not contribute saturated fats nor cholesterol, but they do contribute a good dose of fiber, which is very beneficial. So, it could be said that foods of plant origin rich in proteins are very recommendable. A good option is that 50 percent of the proteins in your diet come from fish, eggs, or white meats; and the other 50 percent from plant foods.

Fats

They constitute one of the most conflictive nutrients after menopause because of the changes we suffer in the lipid profile. In any case, despite being the nutrient with the greatest energy value (1 gram of fat releases 9kcal), fat is essential for health, but in adequate quantities. More than 30–35 percent of a balanced diet's total calories should come from fat. In addition to contributing energy, fats are fundamental for our body because they perform vital metabolic functions: they form part of the cellular membrane, provide essential fatty acids, and are responsible for the transportation of liposoluble vitamins (A, D, E, and K). They also protect us from the cold and strengthen the taste of food. Now, not all fats are equal within this percentage, it is considered that the diet should not contain more than 10 percent of saturated fats, between 6–11 percent of polyunsaturated fatty acids, and the rest monounsaturated fats.

Fats That You Need to Limit

You should limit saturated fats of animal origin that are found in cold cuts, cured cheeses, fatty meats, whole dairy, etc., because an excess will cause you to gain weight and will increase your cardiovascular risk. This type of fat is also found in many packaged foods, in which vegetable fats from palm and coconut are used during their production. With regard to "trans" fats, you already know that they are even more damaging for health. They act in a similar form to saturated fats and are principally found in industrialized foods that contain vegetable fats that have been submitted to a hydrogenation process to solidify unsaturated vegetable oils. Some of the products that contain large quantities of trans fats are margarines, pre-cooked meals, baked goods and commercial cakes, and industrial sauces and fried foods. The best that you can do not only for your weight, but for your health in general, is to completely eliminate this type of food from your diet.

Fats That You Should Include in Your Diet

Unsaturated fats that foods of vegetable origin (except palm and coconut) and fish produce, are beneficial in general. Within this large group, there is distinction between monounsaturated and polyunsaturated fats.

∗ Oleic Acid: Extra Virgin Olive Oil

This oil contains oleic acid (monounsaturated), a good dose of vitamin E, and antioxidant components. It is currently well established that this fat plays an important preventative and therapeutic role in the treatment of heart disease. But what's more, it is proven that having it daily facilitates longevity, slows the appearance of cognitive problems, improves diabetes, and prevents the development of certain tumors, especially those of the breasts and the colon. Additionally, it reduces gastric acid, is an effective laxative, and stimulates the absorption of minerals like calcium.

Numerous studies have also shown that a balanced diet in which virgin olive oil substitutes other less healthy sources of fat diminishes the incidence of obesity. Have it every day (for cooking as well as to dress your dishes), but do not abuse it, because it is very caloric (three tablespoons a day is sufficient).

* Polyunsaturated Fatty Acids: Fish and Nuts

Polyunsaturated omega-3 fatty acids (EPA and DHA) play a fundamental role in the stabilization of cellular membrane and possess beneficial cardiovascular properties. There is no doubt that this type of fat is fundamental for the maintenance of health and wellbeing in the menopausal woman. In addition to helping reduce cholesterol and triglyceride levels in the blood, they have antithrombotic, vasodilatory, and anti-inflammatory activity and contribute to regulating blood pressure. They also actively intervene in the prevention of cancer and improve the effectiveness of antitumor chemotherapy. Studies exist that confirm that omega-3 acids reduce the risk of breast, colon, prostate, and pancreas cancers. What's more, according to a study published in the magazine *British Journal of Nutrition*, omega 3s are related to a lower obesity index. During perimenopause, the hormonal imbalance oftentimes also leads to the appearance of symptoms of depression. In this sense, omega-3 fatty acids contribute to improving this situation, as well as other changes with the cognitive system.

Omega-3 fatty acids are found in fish, above all blue, and in walnuts and flax seeds. Walnuts, in addition to healthy fats, are a source of minerals, fiber, vitamins, and numerous antioxidant substances, which is why it is recommended to have a handful (some 25 grams) every day.

Caveat: Methylmercury

As a consequence of environmental contamination, today it is common to find remains of methylmercury in most fish. This compound is liposoluble and accumulates, above all, in the brain, liver, and kidney. Because of this, having too much blue fish that is contaminated with this substance could principally damage these organs.

The species that tend to accumulate the most elevated quantities are large predators, i.e. those who eat smaller fish. These include the shark, swordfish (emperor), bluefin tuna, and pike. However, smaller fish often contain low levels of mercury, so they do not pose a health risk.

Since eating fish contributes advantages that are much more significant than the disadvantages, you should have fish four times a week (small blue fish, twice). Vary the species you eat, and when it comes time to choose blue fish, always decide on the smaller ones like sardines, anchovies, mackerel, etc. As a rule, remember that the older and bigger the fish, the greater concentration of methylmercury it contains.

Always eat it well-cooked (avoid eating it raw), and remember that the simple techniques like steaming, boiling, and cooking in the oven or on the grill are the most appropriate options. If you also combine the fish with vegetables, you will have a heart healthy, light dish that is rich in fiber, vitamins, and antioxidants, which will be a great help to your health.

Vitamins and Minerals

Apart from the aforementioned nutrients, your diet can also not be missing essential vitamins and minerals. These nutrients do not contribute energy (they are non-caloric), but, although we only need them in small quantities, they are completely indispensable. Without them our cells would not be able to correctly carry out their functions, which is why any vitamin deficiency can seriously damage health.

Since the body itself cannot produce vitamins, you should get them through food (this is why they are called "essential" nutrients). But, since no food that contains them all exists, your diet should be balanced and varied (with foods of all groups and colors) to cover the necessities of these micronutrients.

Fresh fruits, vegetables, and leafy green vegetables are the best source of vitamins and minerals. Whole grains, legumes, and nuts also contain a good and varied quantity. Meanwhile, foods of animal origin, like fish, lean meats, eggs, or fat-free dairy have the trait that among their vitamins is vitamin B12, which only is found in this type of food.

Diet, Yes. Vitamin Supplements, No.

Do not fall into the error of believing that since the lack of vitamins damages health, having them in large quantities will help you to be healthier. It is simply not so. Vitamins are necessary in their exact measurement, not more, nor less.

Studies exist that indicate that the majority of the vitamin supplements offer few or no benefits (except calcium and vitamin D supplements), and in some cases can even be harmful. For example, a study published in the magazine *Archives of Internal Medicine* observed that the use of vitamin and mineral supplements can be associated with a greater risk of premature death, especially in postmenopausal women.

In some specific situations (pregnancy, deficiency states, restrictive diets due to medical reasons, anemia, etc.) these products can be useful, but you should always have them under the control of a doctor. So, do not get carried away by the current tendency to take vitamin supplements to "prevent" a disorder, without the assessment of a professional.

Antioxidants

It is proven that those who consume a diet rich in vegetables protect their health and even improve their physical appearance. In other words, this type of food not only allows you to add more years to your life, but also improves the quality of the remaining years of your life. This effect is due to the numerous antioxidants they contain.

You already saw in the chapter dedicated to skin that the importance of these substances resides in their capacity to block the action of free radicals and the processes of oxidation in the body that harm cells and organs, and consequently deteriorate the body with the passing of time. So, despite the fact that these compounds cannot completely eliminate these processes, they do diminish them. Because of this they are essential to slow the aging process and reduce the risk of developing chronic and degenerative illnesses like heart disease or cancer.

Our body relies on its own antioxidant system to neutralize and eliminate these harmful substances, but much of the time it is not sufficient. Because of this it is essential to count on the extra help of a diet rich in antioxidants.

You can ensure you are consuming a sufficient amount of these substances by increasing fresh fruits, vegetables, and leafy green vegetables in your meals. They are also found in whole grains, legumes, nuts, and virgin olive oil.

Low and Constant: Antioxidant Doses

Antioxidants function effectively in low and constant doses, which is how they are taken through the diet.

Despite the fact that every day more antioxidant supplements are sold, remember that stuffing oneself with this type of product can become counterproductive.

How to Eat Well Without Gaining Weight

Until now you have seen the nutrients and foods that should not be missing from your diet. Now the moment has arrived to establish some simple rules for you to design your diet plan. But first, one piece of advice: get organized.

Many times, not eating well is a result of lack of organization. For this not to occur, the first thing you thing should do is mentally prepare yourself to start feeding yourself healthily and lightly to care for your health and your weight. And dedicate time to organize and plan a weekly menu. Once you have a food plan designed that you are going to follow, make a grocery list, and go to buy it so you have a full fridge. Having a predetermined schedule for meals will also help you to keep your diet healthy, at least in the beginning (you can hang it on a board or on the door of the fridge).

A Complete Diet

A light diet that works without damaging your health must be balanced and complete, which is to say, should provide you the energy and all the nutrients your body needs each day. For this, the trick is in combining all food groups in their adequate measurements.

Throughout the day, you should include five moderate servings of foods rich in complex carbohydrates. This means that, in one meal, two servings of the same type of food should not coincide. You can choose among whole grains, legumes, or starches like potatoes.

You also have to include a moderate serving of some food rich in proteins in at least the three principal meals. You can choose from lean meats, fish, eggs, or legumes. Remember that, if you choose the last ones, you should combine them with whole grains to complete them.

With regard to vegetables, you should count on a minimum of two servings daily, one at midday for lunch (preferably a salad) and another for dinner. In this case, if you eat them raw or cooked simply, the quantity can be abundant. Also include three pieces of fresh fruit every day. You can have them with breakfast, as a dessert, or as a midmorning or afternoon snack.

Among dairy, fat free yogurt is the best option. Have two or three daily. To cook and dress, always use virgin olive oil.

Five Meals a Day

Distribute your diet in five daily meals and do not skip any. Eating lightly and frequently, without letting more than three hours pass between meals, will not only help you manage to maintain the sensation of satiation, but it will also allow you to keep blood sugar levels stable and therefore avoid its drop.

When lots of time passes without eating, your body produces hypoglycemia (low level of blood sugar). This situation produces a lack of energy which is increased by wanting to eat. The result is that you snack in a way that lacks control as soon as the opportunity presents itself.

Fewer Calories, Without Feeling Hungry

After reaching forty years of age, our energy needs diminish 5 percent per decade because our metabolism becomes slower. This translates in our diet having to contribute fewer calories. If you do not keep this fact in mind and you continue consuming the same caloric quantity as before, you will probably gain weight. Remember that the problem is that during perimenopause we have a greater tendency to accumulate pounds on the waist, and that abdominal fat is a cardiovascular risk factor.

Now, the fact that the diet should be lighter does not mean that you have to go hungry; but it does imply that you must prioritize the foods with greater nutritious density (with a high percentage of essential nutrients and few calories). Fortunately, those that have less caloric content tend to be those that contribute a greater quantity of fiber, vitamins, minerals, and antioxidant substances. Because of this, if your diet is rich in this type of food, you will manage to have energy, nourish yourself correctly, and feel satisfied for longer.

More Fresh Foods, Less Pre-Cooked

To lighten your diet, the first thing that you have to do is avoid pre-cooked food. In addition to harmful fats and refined flours, it contains lots of salt and numerous additives that do not do anything to improve your health. For the same reason, there should also not be room in your diet for industrial sauces and dressings, baked goods and cakes, commercial soft drinks, etc.

On the other hand, fresh in-season foods do benefit you. These are the base of any healthy diet, but during the perimenopause transition, it is even more important they constitute the pillar of your diet.

More Fruits and Vegetables

Fresh vegetables as well as fruits should be the principal components of your diet. Apart from their nutritional richness, they hardly contain any fat or calories, so they nourish you while helping you to control your weight.

Always remember that no leafy green plant or fruit is fattening, unless you have them in large quantities (except if you eat them fried or breaded). They tend to be diuretic and purifying, and they produce the sensation of satisfaction because of their richness in water and fiber. This is why they are the first chosen food in diets to lose weight.

Complete Breakfast

Skipping any meal, especially breakfast, is counterproductive for weight loss. Breakfast is very important because it is the first meal that you have after the night's rest and it will allow you to initiate your daily activity with energy and normalcy.

If you do not start the day well, it is likely that at midmorning your energy will begin to fall and your capability for concentration and performance will begin to fail. What's more, soon you will feel a voracious hunger that will push you to eat anything before the midday meal.

It is best to try to have a complete breakfast. A good option consists of having a serving of whole grains, nonfat dairy, and a piece of fresh fruit. If you tend to wake up without feeling hungry, try having a glass of homemade fruit juice or an apple upon getting up. The fruit will help to put the body in motion.

Light Snacks

Having a small, healthy, and light snack in the mid-morning and afternoon is practically essential to ensure you will not be too hungry by the time of the next meal. To soothe the itch of hunger while hardly adding any calories, always choose light and satisfying foods like, for example, fresh seasonal fruit or a fat free yogurt.

Have a Light—but Complete—Dinner

Make sure your dinner is complete, satisfying, and lighter than the midday meal. In this moment of the day it is especially important that you limit fats (above all saturated and trans fats) and that you do not have too many condiments. The reason is to try to facilitate digestion and to not interfere with sleep. In this sense, you should also have dinner early to be able to lie down after digesting.

Include a plate of vegetables, a moderate serving of some protein-filled food, and something else rich in complex carbohydrates. It would be an error to eliminate proteins and complex carbohydrates from this meal because of the argument that your body doesn't need more energy since you are going to sleep. Keep in mind that, although the body uses less, it continues needing glucose to carry out its vital functions. Because of this, what you should do is choose them well and manage the serving.

On the other hand, use dinner to complete the menu of the day, which is to say, prepare it with the light foods that you haven't had throughout the day. For example, if you had a salad and chicken with rice for lunch, you could have a plate of steamed vegetables and a slice of hake with a baked potato for dinner.

Drink Water

Drinking eight glasses of water throughout the day will help you to stay well-hydrated, to avoid the retention of liquids, to dilute and eliminate toxins through urine, and to prevent constipation. What's more, water does not contribute calories (it is not fattening) and, if you have a glass before the meals, it will calm your appetite, so you will avoid eating in excess. Because of this, whenever you have the urge to snack between meals, drink a glass of water because it will help you to control it.

Other light and healthy drinks that you can count on are infusions without sugar, homemade juices and smoothies of fruits and vegetables, or nonfat vegetable broths. But avoid drinking alcoholic beverages, gassy soft drinks, and commercial juices.

Other Advice to Keep in Mind

* Chew Your Food Well

The sensation of satiation tends to be produced twenty minutes after beginning to eat, so if you chew quickly and hurriedly you will end up ingesting up to double or triple the amount of what you really need before your brain sends the signal that you are "full." So, take the necessary time to chew your food well. This way you will better control what you eat and you will feel satisfied when you have eaten enough.

✳ Pay Attention to Flavor and Environment

For your diet to be healthy and help you control your weight, it should be appetizing and enjoyable. In this sense, spices and aromatic herbs are the perfect help so you do not miss dressings or high calorie sauces. With just a small amount, they provide a special touch of flavor and multiply the antioxidant effect of your dishes without adding any calories.

But, in addition to what you eat, it is also important how you eat. For example, whenever you can, eat in company, without hurry, and in a calm and relaxing environment. Keep in mind that conversation slows down a meal, making it more enjoyable, and above all, makes you avoid eating compulsively (since while you speak, you cannot eat).

✳ Avoid Toxins

Neither tobacco nor alcoholic beverages have a place in your plan for better health and wellbeing. Smoking harms you in every way, and with regard to alcoholic beverages, there is also not much good to say. However, red wine and beer are an exception. Both drinks are made through a process of fermentation in which the sugars of the prime materials are converted in alcohol. Consequently, this type of drink, in addition to having low alcohol grade, contains other substances from the foods from which they were made. Red wine contains substances with antioxidant, antithrombotic, and anti-inflammatory properties. Consequently, this drink in moderation contributes to preventing the development of heart disease. What's more, it has anti-inflammatory properties, and a certain protective effect against cognitive deterioration. Beer is also a heart-healthy drink in moderation that can have a positive effect on bone health and other symptoms associated with menopause. To benefit from both drinks you should have them in moderation. Do not drink more than two glasses of red wine or beer a day, if it is not prevented for other reasons.

And If You're Overweight . . .

The diet patterns that you just saw help you to adjust your diet so that you will not have problems during your transition into menopause and your weight will remain under control. And, if you already are overweight, this same pattern will help you lose weight.

There is only one sure way to lose weight efficiently without gaining it back: reducing the calories in your diet and increasing energy expenditure by adapting the regular practice of physical exercise to your habits. Physical activity will also ensure that you do not reduce muscle mass while losing fat, that you improve your toning, and you increase your willpower and sense of wellbeing.

Initially, if you do not suffer from any illness, you will lose weight quickly by decreasing 500kcal a day from what your diet normally contains. The objective you should maintain is to lose weight moderately and gradually. The ideal would be to lose between 4.5 and 9 pounds (2 and 4 kilograms) per month, without losing lean body mass, only fat.

Now, if you have significant excess weight, or you have already tried to lose weight and have been unable to, or you suffer some illness, the best idea is to put yourself in the hands of a specialist who will help you to design an effective plan for you. Do not forget that any hypocaloric diet to lose weight should keep age, fat distribution, and the illness and individual conditions in mind.

Once you have reached your desired weight, if you are of average size and depending on your daily routine, your diet should be made up of 1,600 to 1,800 kcal per day. If you have fewer calories, you could fall in nutritional deficits that could lead health problems down the line and faster weight regain. Regaining weight is very frequent in cases of rapid weight loss, as a result of excessively drastic diets.

Reject Miracle Diets

There are many ways to lose weight, but not all of them are healthy. To lose weight, you should not stop eating or follow unbalanced diets because this can cause more health risks than being overweight.

Following a "miracle diet" to lose weight in a short amount of time will bring you dissatisfaction. This type of plan is characterized by the promise of quick weight loss without effort. You lose weight, but you do so by losing water and muscle mass. You do not eliminate fat, which is what really should happen. What's more, the basal metabolic rate decreases so much that when you abandon the diet, it will produce a very obvious rebound effect. This is why it is so common for people who follow this type of diet to regain the lost pounds (or even more) immediately.

References

Allué, J. *Fitoestrógenos en la menopausia*. Aula de la Farmacia, 2005; 2 (16): 70–78.

Bou, N. *Etapa de cambios*. Farmacia Profesional, 1997; 11 (10): 63–68.

Bris, M. *Fitoterapia en la vida de la mujer*. Madrid: EDIMSA, 2001.

Castelo-Branco, C. *Osteoporosis y menopausia*. Madrid: Médica Panamericana, 2009.

Coloma, J.Ll., Castelo-Branco, C. *Menopausia. Diferentes puntos de vista sobre la terapia hormonal*. Jano, 2009; (1743): 31–34.

Consejo General de Colegios Oficiales de Farmacéuticos. *Climaterio y menopausia*. Panorama Actual del Medicamento, 2009; 33 (326): 862–865.

Cuadrado, C. *La menopausia: algo más que un sofoco*. Madrid: La esfera de los libros, 2007.

Cuadros, J., Llaneza, P., Mateu, S. *Demografía y epidemiología del climaterio en España*. Libro Blanco de la Menopausia en España. Madrid: EMISA, 2000.

De la Gándara, J., Sánchez, J., Díez, M.A., Monje, E. *Influencia de las actitudes, expectativas y creencias en la adaptación a la menopausia*. Anales de Psiquiatría, 2003; 8: 329–336.

De Luis, D.A., Aller, R. *Efecto del consumo de soja sobre la masa ósea en mujeres menopáusicas*. Medicina Clínica, 2012; 138 (2): 60–61.

Durán, M. *Fitoestrógenos*. Revista Ginecología y Obstetricia, 2001; 2 (3): 138–147.

Elorriaga, X., Creus, M. *Menopausia y su tratamiento*. El Farmacéutico, 2004; (315): 64–70.

Fernández, M.V. *Trastornos asociados a la menopausia: alternativas terapéuticas*. Jaén: Formación Alcalá, 2008.

García, C., Repilado, F. *Menopausia*. El Farmacéutico, 2007; (375): 73–74.

García-Franco, A.L., Coello, P.A., Gonzalez, I.del C., et al. *¿Debemos cambiar de actitud sobre el tratamiento hormonal en la mujer posmenopáusica?* Atención Primaria, 2009; 41 (6): 295–297.

Gómez, A.E. *Menopausia. Salud genitourinaria*. Offarm, 2010; 29 (5): 60–66.

Gris, J.M. *Isoflavonas en mujeres menopáusicas*. Medicina Clínica, 2006; 127 (9): 352–356.

Grupo de Trabajo de la Sociedad Española de Investigaciones Óseas y Metabolismo Mineral. *Osteoporosis postmenopáusica. Guía de práctica clínica*. Revista Clínica Española, 2003; 203: 496–506.

Grupo de Trabajo de Menopausia y Posmenopausia. *Guía de práctica clínica sobre la menopausia y posmenopausia*. Barcelona: Sociedad Española de Ginecología y Obstetricia, Asociación Española para el Estudio de la Menopausia, Sociedad Española de Medicina de Familia y Comunitaria y Centro Cochrane Iberoamericano, 2004.

Haas, S., Schiff, I. *Síntomas de déficit de estrógenos*. Menopausia. (Eds. J.W.W. Studd, M. Whitehead). Barcelona: Ancora, 1990; 17–26.

Jáuregui, M.T., Lailla, J.M. *Diagnóstico de la menopausia y sus trastornos asociados*. Jano, 2000; 58 (1345): 59–61.

La menopausia, una etapa de la vida. Barcelona: Associació Catalana de Llevadores, 1996.

Landa, J. *Menopausia*. Atención Primaria, 2002; 30 (7): 458–462.

López, M.T. *Come, disfruta, adelgaza*. Barcelona: Editorial Océano Ámbar, 2011.

López, M.T. *La dieta anticáncer*. Barcelona: Editorial Océano Ámbar, 2011.

López, M.T. *La dieta según las estaciones*. Barcelona: Editorial Océano Ámbar, 2013.

López, M.T., Máñez, C. *Salud natural para la mujer*. Barcelona: Editorial Océano Ámbar, 2008.

Madurga, M. *Cimicifuga racemosa en menopausia y lesiones hepáticas*. Panorama Actual del Medicamento, 2006; 30 (296): 808–810.

Madurga, M. *Nueva información de la agencia española de medicamentos sobre la terapia hormonal de sustitución*. Panorama Actual del Medicamento, 2004; 28 (270): 48–55.

Marzo, M., Alonso, P. *Guía de práctica clínica sobre menopausia y posmenopausia*. Atención Primaria, 2005; 36 (3): 269–272.

Navarro, C., Beltrán, E. *Fitoestrógenos. Posibilidades terapéuticas*. Revista de Fitoterapia, 2000; 1 (3).

Northrup, C. *La sabiduría de la menopausia*. Barcelona: Editorial Urano, 2002.

Olazábal, J.C. *La atención a la mujer menopáusica: un objetivo a desarrollar desde la atención primaria*. Atención Primaria, 2000; 26 (6): 405–414.

Palacios, S. *Calidad de vida relacionada con la salud en la mujer española durante la perimenopausia y posmenopausia. Desarrollo y validación de la Escala Cervantes*. Medicina Clínica, 2004; 122 (6): 205–211.

Pérez, M. *Menopausia. Transición*. Farmacia Profesional, 2002; 16 (9): 88–94.

Pimentel, C. *Alteraciones dermatológicas en la menopausia*. Farmacia Profesional, 2003; 17(9): 84–90.

Plantas medicinales para la menopausia. Madrid: INFITO, 2004.

Rafecas, M. *La alimentación en la menopausia*. Acofar, 2004; (428): 45–47.

Rafecas, M. *La vitamina D y menopausia*. Acofar, 2011; (504): 38–40.

Rafecas, M. *La vitamina K en la menopausia*. Acofar, 2012; (519): 44–45.

Rafecas, M. *Nutrición en menopausia*. Acofar, 2010; (494): 32–34.

Rapado, A. *Salud ósea y calcio en la mujer menopáusica*. Alimentación, Nutrición y Salud, 2000; 7 (1): 6–14.

Rueda, J.R. *Menopausia, frente a los nuevos mitos y la medicalización injustificada*. Atención Primaria, 2006; 22 (supplement 1).

Sánchez, R.M. *Menopausia*. Acofar, 2005; (440): 28–30.

Torrabadella, P. *Menopausia*. El Farmacéutico, 2001; (259): 71–74.